The Ethical

Dr Kamal Kumar Mahawar is a practising medical doctor who has had the opportunity of reflecting on a range of ethical and systematic issues that plague health care in India. He writes regularly on subjects pertaining to Indian health care in *India Medical Times*.

Following his graduation from Calcutta Medical College and post-graduation from Postgraduate Institute of Medical Education and Research, Chandigarh, and University of Liverpool, Dr Mahawar has been working as Consultant General and Bariatric Surgeon with National Health Service (City Hospitals Sunderland NHS Trust), United Kingdom. He is actively involved with research and is the editor of several reputed scientific journals. Dr Mahawar is also the co-founder of science portal WebmedCentral.

FOR, MR. CHAND

WITH BEST COMPLIMENTS

FROM: KAMAL MAHAWAR

The Ethical Doctor

DR KAMAL KUMAR MAHAWAR

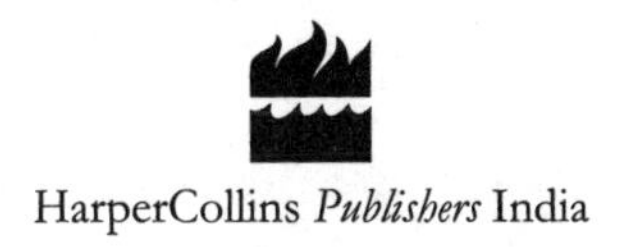

HarperCollins *Publishers* India

First published in India in 2016 by
HarperCollins *Publishers* India

P-ISBN: 978-93-5264-009-6
E-ISBN: 978-93-5264-010-2

2 4 6 8 10 9 7 5 3 1

HarperCollins *Publishers*
A-75, Sector 57, Noida, Uttar Pradesh 201301, India
1 London Bridge Street, London, SE1 9GF, United Kingdom
Hazelton Lanes, 55 Avenue Road, Suite 2900, Toronto, Ontario M5R 3L2
and 1995 Markham Road, Scarborough, Ontario M1B 5M8, Canada
25 Ryde Road, Pymble, Sydney, NSW 2073, Australia
195 Broadway, New York, NY 10007, USA

Typeset in 12.6/16 Linden Hill by
Manipal Digital Systems, Manipal

Printed and bound at
Thomson Press (India) Ltd.

To

My Parents, who sowed the seed

and

My Wife, who is still paying the price

The only thing necessary for the triumph of evil is
for good men to do nothing.

—Edmund Burke

Contents

Author's Note xi
Introduction 1

1 The Concept of an Ethical Doctor 5

2 Cuts and Commissions 25

3 Unnecessary Tests and Treatments 44

4 Drug Companies and Appliance Manufacturers 63

5 Exploitation of the Vulnerable and the Poor 82

6 The Touts 108

7 False Claims 131

8 The Quacks 143

9 The Private Sector 163

10 The Public Sector 183

11 The Regulator 201

12 The Way Forward 225

Appendix 1 247
Appendix 2 250
Acknowledgements 252
Bibliography 255

Author's Note

There are a lot of shortcomings in this world and as an ordinary human being, with only a tiny bit of insight, I am acutely (and painfully) aware of my own. This book does not claim that I am righteous or that the rest of the world is immoral. This book is also not about pointing fingers at any individual or group. In fact, I wholeheartedly believe individuals are rarely wrong; systems often are. I am also old enough, sadly, to know that we are all dealt different cards and we are all trying to make a decent game out of it. We live and work in a society, imbibing its rules and following them. Sometimes, we collectively outgrow a rule that served us perfectly well for centuries. I can give several examples of practices that were the norm for centuries but when we look back today, they seem so obviously wrong. Yet, at the time, these must have been a way of living for people in that era. This book, I would like to think, is a part of the same human journey where we intermittently pause and take stock of the situation and discuss ways to make things better.

Declining values and corrupt practices are eating the heart of Indian society and its institutions. Doctors subscribe to the same value systems. Though this book concentrates on doctors and the delivery of health care in India, there are other functionaries in society—politicians, civil servants, lawyers, businessmen, teachers, and citizens at large—who need to similarly evaluate themselves. Society can only move forward collectively, and so it must be our shared responsibility to engage in such introspection. Not for a moment would I accept that doctors are less ethical or honest than the rest of the populace; nor are they lacking any more in compassion, kindness or any of the other defining human attributes. However, the reality of life is such that over a period of time, each individual is drawn towards the population mean when it comes to values and character.

Sooner or later, somebody is going to point out that I don't myself live and work in India anymore. What right do I then have to talk about India and Indians? Am I not somebody who has run away from this system when I should have tried to stay back and work to improve it? Having obtained free medical education in India, what have I given back to Indian society? I cannot refute any of these allegations, nor do I want to. All I can and will say is that this book is not about me, or what I have contributed to India or the UK—the two countries that have given me all I have in life. That is a very personal matter for me and should be allowed to stay as such.

INTRODUCTION

There must be something about health care that sets it apart from other professions. Others in society do equally, if not more important, jobs; but it is the doctor whom human societies expect the most from and shower with huge respect in return. That is why a doctor falling short of expectations is always news. It is the doctor who has to take an oath on completion of his or her education to follow a code of conduct laid down centuries ago. Some say it is because we deal with human life. But is a lawyer defending somebody facing a death sentence not dealing with human life too? Is a civil servant deciding to give away land owned by poor people to corporates at throwaway prices not dealing with human life? Are teachers not dealing with human life or, for that matter, politicians? What is then so unique about doctors that even societies with remarkable tolerance for unethical and dishonest behaviour want them to act with more compassion and honesty?

The only conclusion I have reached is that it must have something to do with the direct physical pain and suffering that a disease brings. It is as if an illness is an act of god and doctors are the only humans who can help alleviate it. Historically, the air of mystery surrounding health and diseases may also have contributed to placing doctors on a pedestal.

It is my belief that just like a competent law and order machinery is essential for our national well-being, effective health care is essential for our personal and social well-being. Without the former, human societies tend to degenerate into chaos; without the latter, your entire personal life and of those connected to you could be put at risk. Just like a law-abiding state gives you confidence in your dealings within that society, a competent and ethical health care system gives you the confidence to plan your family life.

Patients demand cure and relief. In return, doctors want to earn a respectable livelihood. Patients also expect some compassion and kindness because times of illness are particularly vulnerable times for them. In return, they will give you more respect than other professionals receive. The deal is simple. What then goes wrong with our health care system that this simple deal cannot be delivered? Dysfunctional governance, lack of proper regulations, ineffective planning, self-serving attitudes and, sometimes, overt greed—are some of the many reasons why the health care infrastructure has become infested with a number of unethical practices. As often happens, one mistake snowballs into another and rather than trying to examine the deeper issues and resolve them, every person connected to medicine has invented his or her own 'unique' Indian solution—the quintessential jugaad.

The purpose of this book is to look at these unethical practices that have spread their tentacles deep into the medical profession. Everyone, especially doctors, hates these practices. If there is anybody out there who thinks that doctors indulge in them out of choice, they are terribly and absolutely mistaken. The vast majority of doctors in India want to work ethically and earn an honest livelihood. They want society to recognize their talent, decades of hard work, devotion and sacrifice, and compensate them adequately for it. They want to be provided with the infrastructure for cutting-edge medicine and make a real difference to patients. If a large number of Indian doctors are failing to reach these standards, they cannot alone be at fault. Society and the many institutions in it will need to reflect on it too. That is exactly what this book attempts to do: introspect on behalf of us all.

Rapidly falling moral and ethical standards and the lack of a smoothly functioning 'system' have become hallmarks of many aspects of our lives. How many of us can truly look in the mirror and say that we have been honest and upright all our lives? That we have never taken or given a bribe, that we have been ethical at all times and paid every single paisa of tax.

Individuals are governed by the culture of the herd they live in. If you don't follow the rules, you are not *in* the herd, for the only way to belong is to become like the rest. The closest example of this would be Indian tourists in London. The same people who don't think twice before spitting on the road and throwing litter all around in their own country transform dramatically as soon as they land in London or any other Western city. They know that in this new herd a different set of rules apply. The same principle applies to the medical fraternity in India. Certain norms have found such strong acceptance within the profession that professional bodies and associations are powerless against them and any new entrant must blindly follow them. The same doctors, when they migrate to other countries, behave differently. I know of many Indian doctors settled in the UK and other countries, who take a moral high ground for being upright. But the credit is not theirs for the taking. The credit goes, instead, to the well-grounded systems in place in those societies and their conducive environment. Having said that, every country has its own battles to fight and I don't for a moment believe any individual or group can really take a moral high ground here. Given similar circumstances, all human beings behave in the same way, that is, to first and foremost look after themselves and their own.

I hope this book goes beyond merely listing what is wrong with our health care system, and makes an attempt to understand the reasons underlying the difficulties. I also hope to be able to come up with some practical suggestions. A simplistic enumeration of the problems, though convenient, will not do justice to either patients or health care professionals in India.

Finally, this book certainly does not intend to lay blame on any particular individual or group. Though tempting, such an analysis may prove even more demoralizing for our medical work force which is already struggling with myriad systemic and cultural issues.

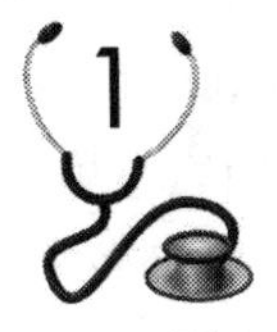

THE CONCEPT OF AN ETHICAL DOCTOR

Ethics is more important than law.

—Anonymous

Freedom is obedience to self-formulated rules.

—Aristotle

'An ethical doctor' is not an abstract concept; the edifice of ethics has been at the heart of the medical profession for as long as the profession itself. Societies have, since time immemorial, expected healers to follow an exemplary code of conduct. That's how an oath invented about 2,500 years ago is very much in use even today. I can't imagine, that back in fifth century BC, Hippocrates would have known that society's basic expectations from the medical profession and its practitioners would remain largely unchanged for so long. Since this oath is the fundamental principle guiding those committed to this profession, it is important that you see what doctors swear by when they don their white coats. In Appendix 1, I have copied both the original Hippocratic Oath and one of its modern versions taken from the website of the largest professional association claiming to represent Indian doctors, the Indian Medical

Association (IMA). At a global level, guidelines for doctors are enshrined in the Declaration of Geneva adopted by the World Medical Association in 1948, which again, I would suggest you go through to get an idea of what the international community expects of its doctors (Appendix 2). As you will no doubt have seen, this declaration has undergone several minor amendments over the last six decades. The point I am trying to make is that though the text has changed somewhat over the last 2, 500 years, even today, doctors in most parts of the world take the oath before entering medical practice.

Why do doctors feel the need to follow a special set of rules over and above those governing civil society? It cannot be because the work of other professionals is any less important than theirs. Nor can it be because society lays down such special rules for doctors. Quite frankly, the public could not care less so long as doctors do their job of healing. My reasoning is that doctors have imposed upon themselves a higher bar of conduct to earn the trust of the patient. Healing, after all, is not just about curing diseases.

All said, the oath is rather symbolic, and practically speaking, doctors in India are governed by a much wider code of conduct—set and regulated by the Medical Council of India (MCI). This code is legally binding on doctors. Take it from me, if this code could be implemented in totality, your doctor will be nothing short of a saint and the medical profession will be cleansed overnight. But the problem is that this set of regulations is not implemented, and as you are about to see, can never be. Simply because, for a legally enforceable code of regulations, it lays down arbitrary rules that are so mindlessly aspirational in nature that they are impossible to implement.

In my opinion, the majority of doctors, not just in India but the world over, will fail this code. Strict implementation of this code would probably bring some much needed discipline into the Indian medical fraternity, but it would cause the eventual destruction of the entire medical edifice. Chances are, you have probably never read this code of ethics. I hadn't, until recently, and I could not believe my eyes when I did. My first reaction was—who dreamt this up? If you don't believe me, as I fully expect you not to, please spend some time reading it yourself. It is freely available on the MCI website. Line after line, it is a comical compilation of rules and values that no mortal doctor can ever dream of adhering to in its entirety. Since we haven't got the time to go over them all, I have selected some particularly interesting sections for you.

1.1.1 *A physician shall uphold the dignity and honour of his profession.*

This is the first line of the code and it sets the tone for the rest of it. There is nothing wrong with this line per se or the principle behind it. But remember, this is not a guidance document teaching doctors how to behave. This is a set of regulations that the MCI decrees you, as a medical professional, have to abide by. It says, 'In exercise of the powers conferred under section 20A read with section 33(m) of the Indian Medical Council Act, 1956 (102 of 1956), the Medical Council of India, with the previous approval of the Central Government, hereby makes the following regulations relating to the Professional Conduct, Etiquette and Ethics for registered medical practitioners.' Courts in India routinely refer to these regulations to settle matters. Hence, it is important that the code is phrased in clear language and that it includes tenets that are enforceable.

Coming back to this specific line, one could come up with any flimsy pretext to accuse a doctor of not upholding the dignity and honour of the profession. Who decides what actions amount to a breach of this regulation? These sentences don't belong in a legal code, which should be dealing in specifics and not woolly language. What the MCI needs to do in this regulation is to state clearly what will be construed as unethical, and then deal with any departures forcefully. In its present form, these regulations are over idealistic and practically impossible to implement.

1.1.2 The prime object of the medical profession is to render service to humanity; reward or financial gain is a subordinate consideration. Who-so-ever chooses this profession assumes the obligation to conduct himself in accordance with its ideals. A physician should be an upright man, instructed in the art of healings. He shall keep himself pure in character and be diligent in caring for the sick; he should be modest, sober, patient, prompt in discharging his duty without anxiety; conducting himself with propriety in his profession and in all the actions of his life.

This is particularly interesting and I am not sure how many of the thousands of students in medical colleges across India are even aware of it. I, for one, did not come to medicine to simply render a service to humanity and nor do I believe did most of the other doctors taking the oath with me. We made a career choice when we were teenagers. Though I thoroughly enjoy looking after my patients and would rather not do anything else, I am not confident I would still want to do my job if I wasn't paid for it. Which world do the writers of this code live in? On the one hand, the courts in India have brought medical practice into the ambit of the Consumer Protection Act; on the other, the regulators expect doctors to work purely for the benefit of humanity.

As you will see later in this book, I am by no means absolving the medical profession, which could do much to set its own house in order, especially in terms of its social responsibility, but to expect all doctors to be saints will never get the desired results. If you read the whole of this paragraph in the code, there are a number of things that have no clear definition and I doubt if these sentences are even required. In a country where we don't have adequate resources to deal conclusively with real criminals, the last thing we want to do is to turn an entire group of professionals into criminals by setting the bar too high. Doing this will only achieve one thing—the real criminals will never be caught and the legal system will keep itself busy with the easily obtainable fruit.

At the same time, I cannot deny the need for the medical profession to do some serious soul-searching. Medicine is not an exact science and far too often, we are helpless in the face of diseases we understand little of. At times, compassion and care is all we can offer. Government doctors in particular have an attitude problem, as their job does not directly depend on the patients and requisite mechanisms for a patient to lodge a complaint against an impolite or rude doctor simply do not exist. What I find more surprising is that even private doctors don't treat patients with the respect and dignity they deserve. Perhaps this is because doctors think politeness will be construed as weakness by patients—a sign of desperation for business. It is also possible that such an attitude comes from lack of knowledge and insecurity. If you are polite, the patient may start asking too many questions, answers to which you may not know. It may even be the lack of time, as a polite conversation with a patient who has thousands of questions may drag on endlessly. Finally, many doctors, just like patients, are fed up of the prevalent second and third opinion culture where patients go from one doctor to the other simply to find out who is better. But can you really blame the patients for not being able to trust the advice they are given, especially when they know it might be inaccurate or dishonest? In a country with hundreds of thousands of quacks and variable standards of education and training, finding a good doctor is no easy task.

1.1.3 *A person obtaining qualification in any other system of Medicine is not allowed to practice Modern system of Medicine in any form.*

Though nobody can put an exact number to it, it is estimated that the number of practising quacks in India is in the range of hundreds of thousands. Strictly speaking, the MCI has no jurisdiction over them; it is a regulator of doctors, not criminals. In my opinion, the issue of quacks is a simple law and order matter and it is the job of the police, not the MCI, to prevent criminals from misguiding and defrauding the gullible public. One has to seriously question this line in a code aimed at medical professionals.

1.2.3 *A Physician should participate in professional meetings as part of Continuing Medical Education programmes, for at least thirty hours every five years, organized by reputed professional academic bodies or any other authorized organizations. The compliance of this requirement shall be informed regularly to Medical Council of India or the State Medical Councils as the case may be.*

This is a reasonable expectation that professionals stay up-to-date with the latest advancements in their field, but what mechanisms are there for such compliance information to be gathered by the MCI or any of its state chapters? I am not aware of any, and I suspect other doctors aren't either. It is another example of a rule that is currently not being enforced and cannot be in the near future.

The MCI has a lot on its plate and sooner or later, it will have to learn to prioritize. The mandated mechanisms to ensure continuance of medical education do not exist in today's India and without a desire or the resources to implement them, the MCI is making a mockery of its own rules.

1.4.1 *Every physician shall display the registration number accorded to him by the State Medical Council / Medical Council of India in his clinic and in all his prescriptions, certificates, money receipts given to his patients.*

1.4.2 *Physicians shall display as suffix to their names only recognized medical degrees or such certificates/diplomas and memberships/honours, which confer professional knowledge or recognizes any exemplary qualification/achievements.*

This is an important regulation with far-reaching implications. However, before it asks practitioners to clearly state their qualifications and registration numbers, the MCI must ensure that it can maintain an accurate register recording information on all medical professionals for cross verification by members of the public and the hospitals. Currently, the MCI does not maintain a database fit for this purpose. There is a lot they can learn, for example, from one that the General Medical Council (GMC) of the UK maintains. It is not only about the search facility, which is grossly immature and raises questions about who designed their website. It is about the database that this search engine enquires. It is not easy to find out from this database where any doctor on the Indian Medical Register is currently working, whether or not they have a specialist qualification, and whether they have been disciplined in the past. I am not sure if the MCI can lay any claim to accuracy here. They maintain a separate list of blacklisted doctors but this does not link with the main register, and if you don't check the two separately, you would not know that the doctor is currently blacklisted. It's not just the MCI website, but government websites in general reflect such abysmally pathetic standards that it is hard to believe that we are actually one of the biggest players in the global software industry.

There is no unique national registration number and the database is not even searchable by registration number. Given this, how does knowing a doctor's registration number help a patient? What is he going to do with that information? Where can he test it for accuracy? It would have been relevant if there was an easily accessible database that patients could interrogate with a smartphone app, whereby they could establish within a few seconds whether the doctor whose office they are sitting in is genuine or a quack. It would have helped to insist that doctors only mention those qualifications that are registered with and approved by the MCI, if a patient could find out on the MCI register whether or not a doctor has actually earned the claimed qualifications, whether or not he is truly a specialist. None of this is currently verifiable and this information gap renders such regulations in the code ineffective.

A quack would not hesitate in flouting this rule or even forging a registration number. It is a different matter altogether that many legitimate doctors, too, exaggerate their qualifications with letters that don't mean much. Once again, here is a regulation that is routinely flouted by a large number of doctors and the MCI has no means of enforcing it.

But with the appropriate supportive and regulatory mechanisms in place, this specific regulation could bring about improvements. But then, the MCI also needs to carry out periodic checks to discipline the defaulters. Without the desire to implement punitive measures, none of these regulations can count for much.

1.5 Use of Generic Names of Drugs: Every physician should, as far as possible, prescribe drugs with generic names and he / she shall ensure that there is a rational prescription and use of drugs.

If you are not a doctor, you may not understand what this means. It means doctors should use the chemical names of drugs and not the commercial brand names. In principle, it is a good idea. If implemented, in one stroke, it could fix the unhealthy nexus between drug companies and doctors as well as reduce the use of hundreds of irrational combinations being vigorously promoted in the market. But in reality, most doctors only use commercial brand names in their prescriptions. I don't know how the MCI can inspire a culture change overnight. Then there are other issues to consider. What will happen to all the combinations that have already been approved? At any rate, I am not sure if people working in pharmacies across the length and the breadth of the country can interpret the generic names correctly. Besides, the quality of drugs can vary significantly depending on the manufacturer, which is probably the most important reason why doctors choose to prescribe reputed brands.

There is another practical problem. If a doctor prescribes a generic drug, how is the pharmacist going to choose one amongst the many available brands in the market for the patient? This will need an almost complete overhaul of drug distribution systems. While the MCI has much bigger issues to deal with, I suggest that it safely ignore generic prescribing, which is something that most countries find difficult to implement.

3.3 *Utmost punctuality should be observed by a physician in making themselves available for consultations.*

This is another example of the kind of trivial MCI regulation could do without. Punctuality is a social attribute and not really the duty of a doctor alone. Can a doctor be punctual if others around him are not? Medical professionals invariably deal with unpredictable events and are not in full control of their time. Moreover, patients who are late, or those with a complex case can delay everyone else in the clinic. Doctors cannot give fixed time slots, as patients themselves can be unpredictable and sometimes don't turn up at all, even when they have an appointment. In such cases, a doctor could lose time and money, without being able to redeem the cost from the patient. Punctuality is a perfect example of values that would be nice to see but that do not really belong in a code that the MCI imposes on doctors universally. Like many other sections in this code of ethics, asking doctors to observe 'utmost punctuality' is impractical and impossible to enforce.

3.4 Statement to Patient after Consultation: 3.4.1 All statements to the patient or his representatives should take place in the presence of the consulting physicians, except as otherwise agreed. The disclosure of the opinion to the patient or his relatives or friends shall rest with the medical attendant.

3.4.2 Differences of opinion should not be divulged unnecessarily but when there is irreconcilable difference of opinion, the circumstances should be frankly and impartially explained to the patient or his relatives or friends. It would be opened to them to seek further advice as they so desire.

3.5 Treatment after Consultation: No decision should restrain the attending physician from making such subsequent variations in the treatment if any unexpected change occurs, but at the next consultation, reasons for the variations should be discussed/explained. The same privilege, with its obligations, belongs to the consultant when sent for in an emergency during the absence of attending physician. The attending physician may prescribe medicine at any time for the patient, whereas the consultant may prescribe only in case of emergency or as an expert when called for.

3.6 Patients Referred to Specialists: When a patient is referred to a specialist by the attending physician, a case summary of the patient should be given to the specialist, who should communicate his opinion in writing to the attending physician.

This section goes into the minutiae of how a doctor should behave when called to give an opinion. Think about it. In a land where doctors stand accused of widespread unethical practices, the regulator seems to be bothered about what someone says and to whom. The code is preoccupied with protecting the interests of the primary physician whereas the MCI needs to be concerned with the interests of the patients and patients alone. It needs to guide and regulate doctors, no doubt, but it certainly does not need to protect them.

4 *Responsibilities of Physicians to Each Other: A physician should consider it a pleasure and privilege to render gratuitous service to all physicians and their immediate family dependents.*

Why should a doctor offer gratuitous services to other doctors? Doctors are usually reasonably well off and can afford to pay for the services they avail. And why should a regulator concern itself with such situations? When most people cannot afford private health care and poor patients are routinely pushed into debt through spiralling health care costs, this code of ethics, instead of talking about how doctors must show some social responsibility, tells them that they should offer free services to each other.

6.1.1 *Soliciting of patients directly or indirectly, by a physician, by a group of physicians or by institutions or organizations is unethical. A physician shall not make use of him / her (or his / her name) as subject of any form or manner of advertising or publicity through any mode either alone or in conjunction with others which is of such a character as to invite attention to him or to his professional position, skill, qualification, achievements, attainments, specialties, appointments, associations, affiliations or honours and/or of such character as would ordinarily result in his self-aggrandizement. A physician shall not give to any person, whether for compensation or otherwise, any approval, recommendation, endorsement, certificate, report or statement with respect of any drug, medicine, nostrum remedy, surgical, or therapeutic article, apparatus or appliance or any commercial product or article with respect of any property, quality or use thereof or any test, demonstration or trial thereof, for use in connection with his name, signature, or photograph in any form or manner of advertising through any mode nor shall he boast of cases, operations, cures or remedies or permit the publication of report thereof through any mode.*

It isn't impossible to comprehend what the MCI is trying to achieve here. Doctors must not get into the business of soliciting business if medicine is to be the noble profession it once was. Modern day reality, though, begs to differ. Medicine is now a business and doctors working in the private sector are in stiff competition with each other and quacks. Survival here depends on a steady stream of patients. Moreover, our tax and legal machinery treats doctors as businesses.

Doctors work in a market environment where continued visibility is important for survival. How else will a patient ever find out about a doctor? What other mechanisms exist in our society to match patients with suitable doctors without patients having to worry about the doctors' competence or doctors worrying about attracting business? In an ideal world, every town and city will have only the required number of doctors; patients will know where these doctors can be found; the number of family doctors as well as specialists will be determined according to the population of the area; and every doctor will be assured of a steady income and inflow of patients. Such an ideal world does not exist. Doctors and hospitals are concentrated in urban areas where they end up fiercely competing with each other for business. At the same time, large parts of rural India have few doctors and hospitals.

Given these underlying factors, most doctors are unable to follow this regulation in spirit. You have to be able to attract some attention if you wish to stay afloat in this market. The MCI cannot truly enforce this regulation as lectures are organized to attract attention and press attention is solicited in the guise of latest medical advancement. I personally feel that the MCI needs to tone down this diktat and simply prohibit active advertising by doctors and hospitals.

Many doctors complain that their peers associated with corporate hospitals have an unfair advantage as hospitals are seemingly exempt from this regulation and corporate hospitals often have large budgets for major marketing campaigns which freelancing practitioners do not.

Now, let us think from the patients' point of view. How do they find out if Doctor A is better or worse than Doctor B? This is a really important question and one that has several offshoots. One could argue whether a patient should really want to know which of the two doctors is better when both are appropriately qualified and licensed to practise. More importantly, can you ever establish that Doctor A is better or worse than Doctor B when doctors themselves don't know where they stand among their peers? Ideally, patients should never have to engage in this exercise. They should be able to go to any of a number of doctors in the area with complete confidence and avail good treatment. Doctors, on the other hand, should never have to worry about attracting work (more commonly addressed as business) and should be able to focus completely on their work. And patients should not need a second opinion to check whether the first doctor gave them accurate advice.

But in the real world doctors have no option but to ensure that they stay on people's radar. They must indulge in activities that attract public attention. This can take many forms like sponsoring a meal for general physicians, or organizing a charitable camp, or developing and promoting new treatments without appropriate ethical safeguards in place, or writing articles for the media, or organizing medical conferences with help from corporates, and so on. This section of the code, in its current form, is disregarded by doctors and unnecessarily makes criminals out of them. It is just one more example of a ruling set down without any practical understanding of how doctors are forced to operate. In my view, until such a day as the other enablers of regulated markets that I have touched upon in different sections of this book are in place, the MCI should just ban overt advertisements and not bother too much with the rest. And when it comes to advertisements, the same rules should apply to both doctors and hospitals.

6.4 *Rebates and Commission:*

6.4.1 *A physician shall not give, solicit or receive nor shall he offer to give, solicit or receive, any gift, gratuity, commission or bonus in consideration of or return for the referring, recommending or procuring of any patient for medical, surgical or other treatment. A physician shall not directly or indirectly, participate in or be a party to act of division, transference, assignment, subordination, rebating, splitting or refunding of any fee for medical, surgical or other treatment.*

There is an entire chapter given to discussing cuts and commissions in this book. Of all the unethical practices destroying the soul of the medical profession in India, this is probably the worst and, apparently, the most widespread. As you can see, in this chapter we are trying to identify those sections of this code that are absolutely pertinent to the profession and must be vigorously defended. This section will stand out in this regard. It is a damaging trend for the medical profession and goes against the inherent ethos of nobility and meritocracy. It is one of those practices that the MCI needs to deal with and deal with forcefully. But it cannot do so until it focusses its efforts on issues that really matter.

7.11 A physician should not contribute to lay press articles and give interviews regarding diseases and treatments which may have the effect of advertising himself or soliciting practices; but is open to write to the lay press under his own name on matters of public health, hygienic living or to deliver public lectures, give talks on the radio/TV/Internet chat for the same purpose and send announcement of the same to the lay press.

Anyone can tell the good intention behind this specific ruling. But how is the MCI going to police it? How will you differentiate an article written in public interest from a promotional one? Is it not up to the press to only publish articles that benefit the masses and identify and discard promotional content as such? For then the task becomes as simple as banning advertisements by doctors. The problem here is that the media is sometimes willing to publish things that don't entirely serve the public good, so as to promote certain individuals or hospitals. And even though the purpose and nature of such content is clearly promotional, it is not openly identified as such. In my view, this is a problem for the media to address, not the MCI. So I would simply get rid of this whole paragraph, as the advertisement section should be sufficient to address the problem.

7.19 *A Physician shall not use touts or agents for procuring patients.*

This is such an important issue that we have devoted a full chapter in this book to talking about it. It would be heartening to see the enforcement of this rule. We must ban the use of agents or touts if we have to protect whatever is left of the sanctity of the medical profession in India.

8.1 *It must be clearly understood that the instances of offences and of professional misconduct which are given above do not constitute and are not intended to constitute a complete list of the infamous acts which calls for disciplinary action, and that by issuing this notice, the Medical Council of India and/or State Medical Councils are in no way precluded from considering and dealing with any other form of professional misconduct on the part of a registered practitioner. Circumstances may and do arise from time to time in relation to which there may occur questions of professional misconduct which do not come within any of these categories. Every care should be taken that the code is not violated in letter or spirit. In such instances, as in all others, the Medical Council of India and/or State Medical Councils have to consider and decide upon the facts brought before the Medical Council of India and/or State Medical Councils.*

The physician should practice methods of healing founded on scientific basis and should not associate professionally with anyone who violates this principle. The honoured ideals of the medical profession imply that the responsibilities of the physician extend not only to individuals but also to society.

And this sums it up. Basically, the whole set of regulations is not enough and the MCI can challenge anybody it likes for any other form of professional misconduct. In other words, if the MCI does not want a particular person or group to belong in the profession, it will always be able to find a number of means to discipline them. No ordinary doctor can possibly comply with all these rambling regulations. And that explains why most doctors choose to ignore the MCI code altogether. Being ambitious is a good thing but in this case, I think the fine line between ambitious and impractical has been crossed. The MCI has limited resources and serves a large country with an immature law and order machinery. It needs to be realistic in its expectations.

Currently, the code is full of sections that are either unnecessary or impossible to implement. Some are even counterproductive and actually achieve an opposite goal. The MCI needs to recognize doctors as professionals expecting to earn a decent living. Yes, in return, they are expected to maintain a minimum basic standard of competence and moral integrity, but asking them to work for the goodness of mankind is not going to achieve it. In fact, if we look at the present day scenario, the effect has been exactly the opposite. The ground realities of the medical profession do not match the MCI's aspirations.

In many areas, this code is redundant and prohibits what is clearly unlawful in the first place. It is like banning the banned. If this code is aimed at doctors, why do they need reminding that quacks should not be practising medicine? That is a matter for the police to handle. Just as the media can decide what is important for public consumption when they publish anything on a topic related to medicine, the MCI needs to understand that it is not here to police everybody in society. The aim of this code is to ensure that doctors maintain a high standard of ethics and if the MCI concentrates only on this aspect of medical practice, it will be much more likely to be successful.

Every institution needs resources and one area where we have failed rather spectacularly is in ensuring that the big public institutions are adequately funded. Yes, money is required for the initial setting up of facilities and it is only natural that at a nascent stage, a substantial state-sponsored or charitable grant would be required. But going forward, can this situation not be changed? Indian colleges, universities and other institutions, despite the significant pool of untapped talent available, struggle to compete globally because they are not self-reliant and remain dependent on state patronage, which also means that they are never free of state interference.

The MCI is a fine example. It is almost entirely state-funded and hence, state-controlled. It does not have the resources it needs to deal with and regulate a large medical work force in such a large country. If the government wants the medical profession to have an effective regulator overseeing it, it needs to allow the MCI the freedom to generate its own revenue and manage its own affairs. I am confident doctors will be willing to pay a reasonable annual registration fee, so long as it is easy to make these payments and they are assured that the money is spent appropriately. Doctors themselves, more than anybody out there, want this profession sorted out and freed from corruption. It is impossible for any doctor to work with dignity and honesty and yet be able to earn a decent, respectable livelihood on par with others who possess similar levels of talent and education. It is up to the MCI to create an environment where these goals become a reality. It is its job, enshrined in the books of law.

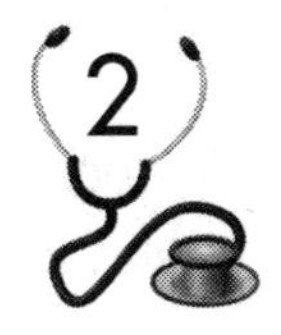

Cuts and Commissions

Doctors get Rs 30–40,000 just for referring a patient for angioplasty.

—Dr Rajendra Malose in the *Indian Express*, Pune, 26 February 2015

All investigations attract a 10–15 per cent kickback to the referring doctor. One day, the marketing executive at this clinic turned up at the hospital with an envelope full of cash—the commission for investigations ordered in the past few months.

—Dr David Berger in *British Medical Journal*

Your doctor refers you to a diagnostic facility, specialist or hospital for some tests. What would you think? That your health demands it. You'd think it's in your best interests; you need the test or the treatment, and the people you are being referred to are the ones best equipped to help you. Presuming that such referrals are only protecting your interests is precisely that—a presumption. In reality, your doctor may have a vested interest in referring you to another doctor or treatment facility—he may earn a proportion of the money you spend on these tests and treatments as commission. This practice in our health care system, when the referee of a patient pays out to the referrer for sending him 'business', is known as 'cut practice', or simply 'cut' or 'referral fee'.

Quite simply, it means doctors have a selfish reason behind sending patients for tests to the diagnostic facility that gives out maximum commissions, or to the specialist who will give them the highest cuts, or to the hospital that will send them maximum referral fees, irrespective of the quality of these services. These financial considerations motivating a doctor pose a strong conflict of interest and the obvious fallout is that a patient can never be completely certain that he actually needs the test or the treatment.

How bad is the situation today? Since the MCI, as we saw in Chapter 1, has explicitly banned fee sharing, such a practice can only go on covertly, without patient knowledge. It is actually a form of corruption, and many believe it to be fairly widespread and an established system in itself, one that even honest doctors get sucked into, eventually. The scale of this practice is probably embodied in a remark made by a professor of cardiology in the *Indian Journal of Medical Ethics*: 'Pernicious as it is, cut practice has come to stay.' Though almost everybody agrees it exists, its exact impact and prevalence has been a matter of some debate. For example, Dr Akash Rajpal of Ekohealth suspects patients end up paying almost 30–50 per cent more than actuals due to this practice. This is higher than an estimate published in the *Indian Journal of Medical Ethics* which states that as much as 20 per cent of the total expenses incurred by the patient are 'transferred' to the general practitioner. Personally, on the basis of my interactions with hundreds of doctors, I think one could safely assume the figure to be somewhere in the range of 20–40 per cent. Naturally, who suffers as a result of this extra cost is obvious, but if you are not sure, a report in the famous British journal, the *Lancet*, quoted

Amar Jesani, editor of the *Indian Journal of Medical Ethics* as saying: 'It's the patient who ends up paying extra money to cover for the kickbacks.'

It is widely held that many doctors earn more from these bribes than from their transparent consultation fees. This, one would think, is absolutely scandalous in a country where millions are pushed into poverty each year simply as a result of expenditure on health care. Bribery and corruption has, sadly, come to define India, and it is clear that our doctors are no less prey to such moral decline.

The reason I have chosen to deal with this—amongst many unethical practices that have over the decades engulfed the medical profession in India—first in this book is the general perception that it is a widespread problem, which causes maximum damage to the credibility of the profession. Almost every single medical practitioner I know confirms that it is a rampant phenomenon, declaring of course in the same breath that they are the only ones around to not indulge in it! The more honest ones have said things like, 'It is impossible to survive without giving commissions, but you can refuse to take it', or a reluctant 'It is the industry norm these days'. It seems to have become standard practice, part of community culture you could say. Like with everything else, once a critical number of people are involved, the others have no choice. You might be unwilling but it's the majority that will decide the rules of the game that you will have to follow sooner or later.

Perception and Reality

Regulators often claim that the practice is confined to a handful of greedy doctors in stark contrast to the popular perception that it is a ubiquitous phenomenon. In a country that tops the global charts when it comes to corruption, where the black economy is bigger than the legitimate economy, there is really no way anybody can put an accurate number to the prevalence of such activities. Most of these transactions take place in cash and short of a massive sting operation undertaken by keen journalists, it would be impossible to know the true extent of corruption involved. Dr Sanjay Nagral, who has written extensively on this topic in the *Indian Journal of Medical Ethics*, has been quoted as saying: 'There is no concrete data on this practice. But a majority of referrals are based on some form of fee splitting.' Even doctors on the ethics committee of the MCI confess that the practice exists.

Rather than arguing about the actual statistics of prevalence (which many people think is close to 100 per cent), to me this is one of those issues where perception matters, even if it is worse than the reality. Perception alone is enough to damage credibility. And for a profession like medicine, where credibility rests almost completely on trust, this perception is doing irreparable damage to the doctor–patient relationship in our country.

'Faith,' it was written outside the chamber of our old family doctor in Kolkata, 'is the first cure'. If Dr Murmuria was alive today, he would have been very disheartened to know that the last couple of decades have seen a near complete erosion of faith in his profession.

This is probably best exemplified in the way patients routinely seek multiple opinions to determine the correct course of action. A patient with high awareness levels and sufficient time on his hands, guided by well-meaning relatives, may then be able to reach the right conclusion, but a less-endowed soul with nobody to hand-hold him, or somebody in need of urgent attention, has little chance. Cut practice is a major contributor to this trust deficit. We must realize that if the reality of cut practice, as the authorities claim, is not as bad as people think it is, our task of fighting it will only become that much easier.

This practice can take one of several forms, all of which mean that a doctor is 'rewarded' for referring a patient to another doctor, diagnostic facility, nursing home or hospital. Cash, cheques (in the guise of professional fee), expensive gifts and dinners, sponsorship to attend conferences, etc., are some of the common rewards. Sometimes, this gratitude is expressed differently. Reciprocal referral amongst doctors is commonplace. For example, a general surgeon and a cardiologist could agree to send each other patients from their respective specialties. It would, of course, be justified if each of them felt that the other was the best in that field, but not if they were simply scratching each other's backs.

Take the example of this doctor I know who works in a big hospital in a metropolitan city. He recently referred a patient to another renowned specialist in the city. A few days later, the commission duly arrived. The commission market works very efficiently and payments are made on time. There is always a lot of honesty in dishonesty. This doctor, however, did not accept the commission, or at least that is what he told me. Instead, he called this surgeon and said, 'I am unable to accept this. I am sure if you referred a patient to me, you wouldn't either.' The commission was politely declined, but a relationship was forged for the future, on a very clear understanding.

It is estimated that some thirty-nine million families are pushed into poverty every year in India, simply as a result of mounting health care expenses incurred. Commissions to doctors account for a significant proportion of that cost and the trust deficit further escalates costs thanks to second and third opinions sought by patients. Cost to society as a whole is much higher if we consider the time wasted in taking these different opinions and making sense of it all. Shouldn't patients just be able to go a doctor, pay a reasonable fee and trust the advice they get? I may be dreaming of a utopian society here, I won't deny it, but it is a practical dream that can be transformed into reality if we all worked towards it with a firm sense of purpose. Such mechanisms do indeed exist in other parts of the world.

Giving commissions to doctors for referring patients ensures that diagnostic facilities have a steady stream of patients. What started as an additional incentive to doctors by a clever player in the field has now become the industry norm. As a result, doctors no longer need to refer patients to a particular facility, as commission can be expected from every single laboratory in the area. The advantage of any marketing innovation lasts only as long as the competitors take to figure it out, forcing the players to innovate further to survive. The competitive advantage that any laboratory or specialist may once have had is now long lost. Owners of diagnostic facilities today have little choice as all players give out commissions and local doctors refuse to send patients (or even accept the reports issued by the diagnostic facility as accurate) without this cut. A pathologist in Bengaluru wrote in the *Indian Journal of Medical Ethics* that he is routinely asked, 'How much do you offer? The going rate is 25 per cent.' Doctors involved in diagnostic work, like radiologists, biochemists, pathologists, microbiologists and so on suffer the most as they have no direct contact with patients and are dependent on other clinicians for work.

What do you suspect would happen if diagnostic facilities didn't have to pay out these commissions? The tests would become cheaper. Twice in the recent past I got indirect proof of this. Last year, one of my friends needed an MRI done on his knee. He was advised by a third friend of ours, a practicing orthopaedic surgeon, that if he wanted a discount, he should claim to be a self-referral, not mention the name of any referring doctor and ask for a discount. My friend did precisely that and obtained 30 per cent discount. In another instance, an advertisement was aired on a radio channel in New Delhi in June 2014, where the voice claimed to be able to get you up to 50 per cent discount if you routed the tests through them (rather than the doctors). In both instances, diagnostic facilities showed their willingness to pass on the benefits to the consumer if there weren't any intermediary doctors to deal with.

I have heard of multiple cases where the referrer will inform the referee which tests and treatments should be recommended based on what the patient can afford. Now if that sounds like arranged loot, that is exactly what it is. Take the example of this quack from a village who showed up with a patient at the clinic of a doctor I know, and said, 'He knows that he will need a CT scan.' It is also common for radiologists to be asked to confirm the 'provisional diagnosis' so that the surgeon can safely proceed with the operation. The saddest part is that most doctors are not even shy about narrating these stories because everybody believes everyone is in it.

Specialists find it impossible to establish themselves without support from their colleagues in general practice. Life is harder when you have just qualified and have a family to feed. No matter how good you are, you need your general practitioner colleagues to back up your credentials in front of the patients. In this situation, you become the biggest surgeon in town if you give out the biggest cuts to the general practitioners. If you are 'not so good' or a new surgeon in the area, you have to work harder.

So, the next time your doctor tells you about a certain Dr X being the biggest surgeon in town, you should consider asking how your doctor knows that is so. It is simply not possible to carry out evidence-based comparison of the performance results of doctors in most countries. Irrespective of the accuracy, the proclaimed results of these comparative assessments are self-fulfilling prophecies and, from the point of view of a specialist, certainly worth the investment. Moreover, if specialists get the patient first, they will expect the same benefit for referring to other specialists, laboratories or hospitals. So a perverse system is born where one who gets the patient first, benefits the most. Unsurprisingly, this has led to a race to seek patient attention, and that lies at the bottom of a number of aggressive and sometimes unethical marketing practices, discussed elsewhere in this book. Patients have become commodities in this marketplace. They can be, and are, routinely exchanged for money.

Marketing Executives

Many private hospitals hire an army of relationship managers solely for the purpose of organizing 'cuts'. The *Lancet* recently reported that 'many hospitals and clinics routinely issue cheques to doctors under sanitized labels such as "professional fee" to encourage them to recommend their services to their patients.'

Allegedly, the expenses come out of their marketing budgets, and can hence be adjusted against income as necessary business expenses. These marketing executives are very powerful people in private hospitals across the country; every specialist working in big private nursing homes and hospitals knows not to get on their wrong side. You can refuse to cooperate with them, but at your own peril.

There is no denying the fact that setting up a hospital is an expensive undertaking with regular fixed outgoings. You need patients on a regular basis to avoid incurring losses, and the only people who make it possible for you are general practitioners. I recently overheard a conversation between the owner of a private hospital and his marketing head: 'Send everybody who is sending business of more than 20 lakh to Thailand.' Somebody else I met recently boasted of successfully turning around a failing hospital; all he had to do was put in place an efficient marketing team. These are common stories and not isolated examples. And so I couldn't help agree when a prominent newspaper recently quoted a doctor as saying, 'Every [hospital] in the industry indulges in this practice.'

There is widespread recognition that in order to survive, a private hospital must have arrangements with lots of general practitioners. And since everybody is in it, the relative advantage that the first hospital to come up with this innovative idea may have had has long ceased to exist. This is a typical case of how distorted unregulated markets function. Eventually, competing players kill each other and they all lose out. This is precisely what happened to the banking industry in the Western world recently with subprime mortgages. Banks were in a race to give housing mortgages to more and more low-worth clients, creating a vicious circle, a housing price bubble and a need for an even lower quality mortgage product to fund that bubble, until, of course, the bubble burst. Some of the biggest names in American banking history disappeared almost overnight. It is up to us to draw lessons from these events and put corrective mechanisms in place, or else we will see more of these cataclysmic examples of human failure. Human beings are competitive by nature; it is the responsibility of collective society to ensure that competition takes us all to a better place.

Targets

Some private hospitals set targets for their consultants where continued practising privileges depend on achievement of a certain turnover. What do you think these doctors then have to do to meet these targets? Won't they be more likely to request unnecessary diagnostic tests or offer higher cuts to general practitioners?

It does seem as if private hospitals have a lot to answer for. What remains unclear though is whether private hospitals, accounting for a miniscule fraction of the quantum of health care provided in the country, are the main cause of the problem or are simply responding to the demands of an unregulated market. After all, private hospitals as an entity couldn't have single-handedly altered the mind-set and culture of the entire profession. We will, later in the chapter, analyse forces that could have weakened the resolve of the profession to stay true to its original ethical and noble foundations.

At the societal level, incentivizing and respecting a behaviour usually encourages it. If we respect wealth, irrespective of how it is obtained, and give it a social status, why wouldn't everyone seek it by hook or by crook? Wealth brings you respect and the tag of being 'successful' in society. One lacking wealth, no matter how deserving, is labelled a 'failure'. In a society where honesty is considered a weakness and not respected, why would anybody aspire to be honest? These are some of the issues that people in general, and not just doctors, need to examine.

In a scenario where the end is all that matters, I wasn't really surprised when I heard that apparently, many specialists maintain advanced accounts with general practitioners to secure a steady inflow of patients. For example, if the commission for referring one patient is Rs 10,000, then the specialist will give Rs 50,000 in advance to the general practitioner, as if to *buy* five patients, and these accounts are topped up as and when necessary. I do not think it is possible for the medical profession to stoop lower than this, but at the rate we are going, I will most certainly be proved wrong. What does the general practitioner then have to do to ensure this steady supply of patients? Will this become the standard of cut practice tomorrow? And what's next? I leave you to ponder over these questions.

Public sector doctors, though much more transparent in their dealings than their private counterparts, cannot be completely exonerated, when it comes to cut practice. They are known to refer patients out to private facilities, sometimes to the ones they own themselves (self-referral). I personally know a surgeon in a government medical college who used to offer operations privately—for a fee of course—for patients coming to him in medical college, because his hospital theatre slots were always full. Many government hospitals lack facilities to carry out basic diagnostic tests. Patients have to be referred out to private facilities, of course, with an expectation of some benefits in return. In particular, I remember my days as a postgraduate student in surgery, when representatives from a local diagnostic centre would offer us incentive to send them our patients for CT scans whenever the hospital scanner was out of order. How did these people find out every time our scanner was out of order is beyond my grasp. The cynic in me did sometimes wonder though, whether these private players had a role to play in the periodic malfunctioning of our scanners...

It is worth mulling over the fate of specialists who start off as honest and upright doctors. For you to demonstrate that you are a good surgeon, you need to treat some patients first. In the early years of your career, referrals are the only way to get patients. If you don't follow the rules of the market, you won't have any referrals, and you won't survive. It's a simple fact of life which many young doctors learn very quickly. Not giving commissions is not a viable option at the beginning of your career. Later in life, when you are established and can manage without it, your resistance to this practice has died and you've got used to it. Even if you did suddenly want to stop, wouldn't it look odd to take a high moral ground after years of happy indulgence?

Though it is little consolation, the problem is not confined to India alone and can be seen elsewhere. In the United States of America, where, the majority of health care is delivered privately, there's a similar problem, albeit probably on a much smaller scale. Physicians there have been accused of referring patients to services they have a financial stake in. There is evidence that a high proportion of such self-referrals are judged to be clinically inappropriate by independent medical experts. Hospitals in USA are known to incentivize clinicians to keep patients in hospitals for as long as their insurance limits allow.

Even in the public sector National Health Service of the UK, where doctors maintain some of the highest ethical standards in the world, there is talk of 'supply-induced demand'. It implies that procedures ordered by doctors aren't always strictly necessary and the desire to perform them on extra 'initiative' lists for an extra fee may play a role. This practice seems to have become commoner since the introduction of the latest payment mechanisms ('payment by results'), where hospitals are paid according to the number of procedures they carry out. Commissions seem rife in Dubai, and they have also been reported in Singapore and Malta. The medical tourism industry has also been widely criticized for it. Commissions and cut practice happen elsewhere in the world too, but it is the scale of this practice in India that is worrisome. Whereas in other countries, it seems to be confined to a few doctors, here it appears to have become part of the system—a system that individual doctors are powerless against.

While we need to start understanding the causes and explore potential solutions to the problem of cut practice, it is worth remembering that there are doctors out there working completely ethically and professionally. I personally know of a few who, instead of taking commissions, ask diagnostic centres to give discounts to their patients. Such doctors may not be too many in sight, but they are there and they form the backbone of this profession. One such doctor I heard of recently, in Maharashtra, is suing a diagnostic facility for allegedly sending him a cheque (in the guise of professional fee) for referring a patient for a scan.

One bad fish is enough to destroy the whole pond. Why is one good fish not sufficient to cleanse it? Even nature aids the fall and resists the rise.

Business Ethos and a Noble Profession

Indian health care is one of the fastest growing sectors in the economy, growing at a compounded annual growth rate of 15 per cent year on year. The private sector, which constitutes nearly 75 per cent of the total health care infrastructure in the country, accounts for most of this growth. Private funding has brought many benefits, but at the same time it has transformed health care into an industry where individual businesses, many of which are owned by doctors, focus entirely on maximizing profits. How can generating profits be a bad thing for any business? It cannot be, but that is not the question. The question is whether we really want to run our health care like a business. Currently, our approach seems somewhat inconsistent. On one hand, we are encouraging massive corporatization of health, but on the other, we complain when hospitals behave like corporates. It is time for us to take a clear stand as a society.

Industrialization, corporatization and massive growth of the private sector has also influenced how doctors view their own role in society; many of them no longer identify with the tag of a noble profession and the altruistic sentiments of serving humanity. Some doctors feel that bringing medicine under the fold of the Consumer Protection Act has further constricted the character of their relationship with patients. A consumer, they argue, cannot be the beneficiary of an altruistic service. It should have been possible for us to prevent a patient from becoming a consumer by keeping the courts out and strengthening the self-regulatory and external regulatory mechanisms. We took a different route, and the result is there for all to see. A wrong, I believe, was yet again corrected by another wrong.

Unequal Distribution

An unequal distribution of resources, with relative concentration of medical professionals, diagnostic services and hospitals in urban areas, catering to the very few who can afford them, leads to excessive competition for patients in these areas and an almost complete lack of services in the rural areas. For general practitioners, it drives down the genuine transparent fees they are able to charge and acts as a catalyst for them to look for an easy, alternative source of revenue. For specialist doctors and hospitals, it means aggressively competing for a small number of patients. You now have a perfect match—a group of people who are desperate for extra cash, and another group of people who are happy to provide it, to get patients in return. Connect the two groups and cut practice is born.

A leading doctor in Delhi was quoted by a respected medical journal as saying, 'Out of some seventeen million inhabitants of Delhi, barely a million can dream of getting treated at a private hospital. So all the hospitals are vying for patients from that small percentage of people. If they're not going to use kickbacks, they won't stay in business.' Let us ponder this further. Does giving kickbacks suddenly increase the number of people who can afford this care? Of course it doesn't. Increasing the cost actually reduces the number of people who can afford the services. The choice is ours. We can either go down the vicious cycle of cuts, increasing health care costs and reducing the number of people who can afford it; or get rid of cuts, make health care affordable for more people, and improve our own prospects in return in an ethical manner.

Currently, our actions are defeating our own objectives. The fundamental question as always for each doctor in India is—what will happen if everyone does what I do? This is not just a question for doctors to think about though. How many ordinary people in our society can genuinely claim to have reflected on these lines? Let us not forget—doctors live and breathe in the same society as you and I. They live by the same values and aspire to the same ideals.

The Greed

A practice that may possibly have started as a correction to some of the aberrations in the health care system has now become a standard method for doctors to maximize revenue, and this has to be considered the dominant cause in our analysis of this practice. For example, if the practice was confined to some newly qualified specialists trying to build repute, it might be somewhat understandable (though still not justified), but when you see even the eminent established ones indulging in it simply to earn more money, one has to suspect other motives. Every cardiologist wants to become the best cardiologist in town and the quickest way (for the right ways often take longer) to achieve that status is to indulge in cut practice. When a doctor sends you a patient, he will certainly need to convince the patient that you are the best in town in what you do. Your strengths will be magnified and weaknesses downplayed. You become a star overnight.

The idea that greed may be playing a vital role is further reinforced if you just look around. The majority of doctors seem to be doing rather well, financially, and most people would find it difficult to accept that doctors are not being rewarded fairly by society. Most doctors are very well off; some have their own nursing homes, even hospitals. How is it possible for honest professionals, demanding only their fair share from society, to earn that much? Even if one presumed for a moment that they weren't earning a lot, might that be because India is a developing country and doctors can't expect a quality of life and compensation much better than the rest of the population? The vast majority of doctors are only graduates, although they spend longer in education than others, and one would argue that for a graduate, their compensation is adequate. Those amongst them who qualify for specialist training through competitive examinations spend longer periods in training, typically work in secondary or tertiary care centres, and attract better remuneration.

The Road Ahead

Irrespective of the underlying reasons and moral justifications, there is little doubt that cut practice increases the cost of health care and seriously undermines patient confidence and trust in our health care standards. Ideally, referral to another doctor, diagnostic facility or hospital should be determined solely on the basis of their ability to help the patient, and not on their ability to pay cuts. The truth, however, is that doctors have no way of telling the good specialist, diagnostic facility, hospitals, etc., from the not-so-good ones, as the data to reach those conclusions is simply not available, and the decision therefore is always arbitrary. We will discuss elsewhere in this book if it is possible to come up with benchmark numbers that can make this process of identifying the good from the bad a bit more robust.

Adequate Compensation

Not paying people enough is the surest way to promote dishonest behaviour. As a society, we must understand that if we expect doctors to work honestly and ethically, we have to reward them adequately in financial terms. Though what constitutes reasonable compensation is arbitrary, it is not impossible to agree on a fee range for consultations and procedures in different geographical areas and specialties. These fee ranges should be clearly set by the regulatory authorities and doctors should not be allowed to charge more or less than that. Currently, fees vary widely as they have been left to the markets, and aberrations on both sides are commonplace. A bottomless pit encourages people to kill competition by lowering the prices and then supplementing income through unfair means. A limitless ceiling leaves spare money that can then be used to give out cuts.

Legalization of Cut Practice

Another radical suggestion sometimes put forward is legalization of cut practice. The idea does have some merits and is well worth examining. It is not vastly dissimilar to the strategy of legalization of banned substances (like cannabis) in many counties. Such an approach takes a pragmatic view of legal enforcement and provides a seal of legal (though perhaps not moral) acceptability to somewhat questionable human behaviour. After all, why should your doctor take the trouble of finding out an acceptable specialist for you in town, explain everything to you, liaise with the specialist, and ensure overall that you get good care, for the peanuts he is paid as 'consultation fee'? If legalized, a referral fee could be paid in a transparent fashion and it will compensate the doctor for the time and effort spent in protecting your interests. This would be a wonderful idea, if only officially rewarding the practice of referral did not run the risk of encouraging even more unnecessary hospital admissions and operations. This strategy is only likely to work well with strong supervisory safeguards in place.

Experience teaches us that it is challenging for any regulatory framework to overcome the hurdles of inefficiency, bureaucracy and corruption. On a more philosophical note, legalizing criminal tendencies may act as an enabler in the short term by freeing up our criminal justice system to deal with more sinister challenges, but in the longer term, it can by itself determine our moral values and alter our notions of what is acceptable behaviour. Legalization will pose a further ethical dilemma of overburdening the sickest in society with referral fees on top of all the other necessary expenses that they must incur.

Cut practice has to stop, and believe it or not, hospitals, laboratories and even doctors want the practice to come to an end. But nobody can do it in isolation for fear of losing out. This is where collective action on behalf of society is required. All the MCI needs to do is to conduct a few robust covert investigations and deal with the culprits decisively—by that I mean, give out a punishment that will deter others from indulging in similar malpractices. Punishing a few is all that is required to see lasting changes.

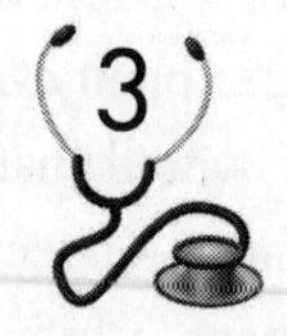

Unnecessary Tests and Treatments

People say that in some places, there are whole districts without uteruses. It seems that private doctors see this as an opportunity to make a fast buck. They're making money on ailments which could be treated in a simpler, less invasive way.

—BBC World Service, Rajasthan, India, 6 February 2013

Most doctors tend to scare the patient into accepting the 'only' option available. With the doctor getting a 'cut' out of the cost of the stents used, there is a direct conflict of interest in the treatment involved.

—*Afternoon*, 30 June 2014

A physician told of pathologists pleasing referring doctors by giving false reports, such as labelling healthy patients as having diabetes so that they are dependent on the referring doctor for life.

—Dr Arun Gadre in *British Medical Journal*

The practice of medicine stands at the cusp of two worlds—science and art, the physical and the metaphysical. Over the last few decades, the pendulum has swung significantly towards science. With the ever-increasing availability of diagnostic tools, clinicians no longer need to spend hours talking to patients or feeling their abdomen to look for subtle clues. An evolving array of blood tests and scans has enriched our ability to understand aberrations in human physiology and anatomy in fine detail. Patients too know that these tests improve the accuracy of the diagnosis and treatment. So much so that many patients today are not reassured without the certainty of a test. As a result, doctors want more and more tests done and patients are willingly undergoing them, sometimes even demanding them. Everybody is happy. More accurate treatment is administered and patients are visibly getting better.

There is a slight problem though. These tests come with an attached financial burden, which translates into increased health care expenses. Since, in India, most health care costs are borne by individuals, this strains finite family budgets. Higher health care costs also mean that the benefits of modern medicine do not reach a large section of the population. Given that India is a developing nation, I would say it is our moral responsibility, as doctors, to think of ways to contain health care costs. We bear the responsibility of using these tests judiciously and appropriately. Yet, despite this responsibility resting on us, the use of diagnostic tests is rapidly increasing, and not just here. It is a universal phenomenon driven by a number of factors.

Local Guidelines and Indian Specialty Advisory Groups

Patients hate uncertainty and want clear answers. For good reason, they want doctors to be accurate and correct every single time. Doctors are aware that they need to use diagnostic tests liberally to be able to deliver on these expectations and to justify their actions to independent observers. Desire for perfection and fear of litigation are two major contributory factors to the dramatic increase in use of diagnostic tests seen in recent years across the world. The problem is further compounded by the fact that doctors work in a fiercely competitive market, where even a slight delay in diagnosis and cure may result in loss of business.

There is another issue to consider. It is impossible for individual doctors, especially general practitioners, to keep pace with all the latest developments in medical science. In a difficult clinical situation, where it might be possible for a very well-read doctor to reach an appropriate conclusion with just one or two tests, a less informed doctor will generally end up requesting a number of irrelevant tests and still struggle to get to the right place. The same applies to treatment. Competent, well-trained doctors use few, targeted medicines whereas the unsure ones end up prescribing a cocktail of drugs to cover all possibilities. Lack of adequate knowledge can also lead to unnecessary hospitalization, procedures and operations. We will discuss elsewhere in this book how standards of medical education and training are variable across the country and, in some places, frankly pathetic.

Individual doctors need support and guidance in their day-to-day practice. We need to come up with acceptable local algorithms and guidelines for diagnoses of common symptoms and diseases that health care professionals can use without fear of losing patient confidence. Yet, this is one area where the health care system in the country has failed most abysmally, despite there being hundreds of professional associations.

This is probably because office, bearers in these associations are not able to place the interest of the patients above that of the members they represent. As a result, these associations rarely command much respect in society and possess little leverage with the government or the media. In an ideal world, the chief goal of professional societies would be to develop and disseminate best practice guidelines. One mustn't, however, forget that office-bearers in these associations are democratically elected by the membership and not by the patients. So it isn't difficult to understand whom they feel answerable to and whose interests these associations chiefly concern themselves with. Though there are some well-meaning clinical guidelines issued by professional associations, they are few and far between.

These associations organize their annual conferences with much fanfare where some knowledge-sharing does take place but the emphasis is on luxury accommodation, food, and who is delivering a talk in which time slot and who will moderate. By and large, they do not come up with any policy statement that can influence training, education or patient care. When they do come up with a consensus statement or guideline, it is usually not for the above purposes or for the progress of science, but to promote the interests of their members. I admit that these are sweeping generalizations and unlikely to be completely true, but hopefully I have been able to provide an indication of how the associations work.

To address this problem, we need professional bodies supported and recognized by the government and public. Such bodies should have representation from a variety of stakeholders (for example, international as well as national experts, the wider public, patient groups, the government, public sector hospitals, private sector hospitals, etc.) and be independent of all influences. Their sole job should be to take into account all local factors and issue clinical guidelines on important topics. Such Specialty Advisory Groups will be able to develop their specialties in line with the needs and expectations of the public, which our professional associations have been unable to do. These advisory groups would exclusively represent patient interests, and not those of the profession or any other group. They will also ensure that our health care remains affordable and relevant to realities on the ground.

Once these groups are in place, the public and the government should listen to them on important policy matters. The government needs to realize that devolving health care policy decisions in this manner, and then of course holding these advisory groups accountable, is the only way to develop a truly effective national health care system. Before you think I am digressing, the reason I am bringing it all up here is that such guidelines on the use of diagnostic tests and treatment of common conditions would reduce the use of unnecessary tests and treatment, thereby enhancing trust in the doctor–patient relationship. For Indian guidelines, one would expect these advisory groups to take into account Indian realities and not simply replicate Western guidelines. In many areas, there may be a genuine lack of relevant research. These areas should be systematically identified and local research encouraged. These guidelines will no doubt need to be mindful of what patients can afford and of the working circumstances of doctors. I would even suggest that we come up with different guidelines for different clinical settings and patient groups, recognizing that a surgeon dealing with a rich patient in a corporate hospital in Delhi faces challenges, different to one looking after a farmer in a remote town in Bihar.

Screening and Treatment of Healthy People

If you live in Delhi and listen to the radio, you must have heard these adverts from a famous local diagnostic facility—how you must have a number of blood tests carried out every so often to maintain good health. I am not sure if there is any scientific evidence behind this. One does wonder where the advertising regulator is and what rules apply to diagnostic facilities when they make such scientifically questionable claims. India is perhaps unique, in that any individual can go to any diagnostic centre and get any test done. Some tests such as Xrays and CT scans may even have harmful physical consequences. Certain others like positive tests for HIV (AIDS virus) or cancers may have adverse psychological and social consequences. Whether or not you as a patient can interpret a positive or a negative result, you are being encouraged to undergo whole body checks every now and then to ensure you stay fit! Now, here is my opinion as a doctor, and one that I think most doctors in the world would endorse—*you don't need tests to stay fit*. What you need is to follow a healthy lifestyle, live in a clean environment, take sensible precautions, and see your doctor when you have any problem. Not only can unnecessary tests cause direct financial, mental and physical damage, they can also lead to fraudulently wrong reports, unnecessary and sometimes dangerous treatment, and inevitable significant increases in health care costs.

The same is true of the custom of routine health checks being vigorously promoted by many corporate hospitals. As a patient, you will think this is a good idea. You go to a doctor. They examine you and conduct tests, diagnose disease at an early stage, and you stay healthy. However, what you may not know is that the evidence for such routine health checks is not undisputed. Many of the diseases identified in these checks may never cause any significant harm to you whereas the adverse consequences of additional tests and treatment they inevitably demand are real. In addition to a significant financial burden on the health care systems and psychological distress to the individuals, routine health checks may not even translate into improved health outcomes.

Screening of asymptomatic individuals is a significant issue that policy makers and professionals need to examine in some depth. The purpose of all screening is to diagnose diseases at an early stage to improve treatment outcomes. Though screening is routinely recommended for many diseases in Western countries, we lack studies establishing their benefits in the Indian context. This is one of those areas where data cannot be directly extrapolated (not that any data can ever be directly extrapolated across populations), as there are significant differences in lifespan of individuals, genetic makeup and ability of health care systems to cope. There is a lot that India needs to fix in its health care scenario before we start screening normal individuals for diseases. Now, I am not suggesting a blanket ban on all screening in India. What I am trying to argue for is that we make a convincing case for any screening and also define the population to which it will be applicable.

The Indian population is a very heterogeneous mix and one of the responsibilities that fall to the planners and the professionals is to come up with different solutions that suit different groups.

Moreover, health care resources are finite and societies must decide for themselves how they wish to use them. Screening has significant cost implications for both publicly-funded and insurance-funded health care and usually ends up making health care more expensive for everyone. It may be that we recommend screening only for self-funded individuals who can bear the costs not just of the screening but also of the (usually negative) tests and treatments that follow. Such an approach will also act as a future cohort in studying the benefits of screening for the Indian population.

No two individuals are the same. This fact doesn't prevent some doctors from treating accepted variations in physiological parameters as diseases. Prescriptions for tonics for thin individuals, nutritional supplements for tiredness, treatment of low blood pressure, medication for slightly high cholesterol—all fall in this category. What can be corrected with simple dietary advice is often treated with a tablet. If you have some cold and cough, irrespective of the fact that a vast majority of these are viral infections, a large number of doctors will prescribe antibiotics. Part of this comes down to patient psyche—some patients only value a doctor who prescribes a few tablets. Medical advice itself often counts for nothing. The medical community has responded, not by launching mass health education campaigns, but by giving in to the public clamour for capsules.

There is another angle to this debate. Doctors are working in a market. If patients do not get quick relief, they will go to somebody else. Doctors often treat a number of conditions simultaneously, to avoid missing any. If you visit a doctor with fever, your doctor will often treat you for a number of common causes simultaneously. Furthermore, many diseases are self-limiting and don't need any specific treatment. Doctors wouldn't tell patients this for fear of losing business. Hence, they prescribe symptomatic treatment and proclaim a cure while nature takes care of the disease.

Practising systematic and evidence-based medicine, in absence of respected local guidelines that both patients and doctors can trust, is a luxury that very few doctors can afford. Here, if a patient is not cured in a couple of days, he changes the doctor, and doctors are continually worried about surviving in a tough marketplace rather than honing their professional and academic skills. We must understand that medicine is both a science and an art. It often takes time to get to the correct diagnosis and doctors usually develop safe algorithms in their areas of practice. If you, the patient, don't accept this, you will indirectly end up pressurizing your doctor to treat you for all possibilities. This causes real harm and inflates health care bills.

Nevertheless, patients are not entirely stupid and it is important to understand the rationale underlying observed patient behaviour. In a country where it can be difficult to differentiate quacks from doctors; where fresh pass-out doctors are given the licence to practice without any further training; where unethical medical practices are rampant and the medical regulator itself stands accused of corruption, how can any patient really be sure that correct treatment is being given? Trust lies at the rock bottom of the doctor–patient relationship and that is the fundamental issue in this analysis. A series of bold and determined initiatives will be required to restore that trust.

Medical Corruption

Now that we have dealt with some of the more legitimate reasons for unnecessary tests and treatment, we can enter the territory of the illegitimate. What we have discussed so far are somewhat global challenges, faced by doctors and patients universally, in a continually changing social spectrum. But contemporary Indian medical practice is different, and doctors here stand accused of widespread corruption. Unnecessary tests, hospital admission, procedures and operations have, unfortunately, become a source of easy money for many doctors, diagnostic centres, hospitals and nursing homes. It is now common knowledge that some doctors prey on the patients' fear of diseases to recommend tests and treatments that are wholly unnecessary.

These are tests and treatments performed entirely for the financial gain of doctors and hospitals, and may actually harm the patients. This is in addition to the existing burden of expenses that pushes families into poverty, making health care unaffordable for millions, with increased insurance premiums for those with insurance cover, and erosion of confidence in the medical profession as a whole.

Take this case for example. A forty-year-old lady goes to her family doctor for some pain in her abdomen. The doctor organizes a number of tests including ultrasound and endoscopy to find out the cause. The ultrasound scan shows that the lady has stones in her gallbladder and the doctor recommends surgery for this lady. Referral to a surgeon is duly made and the operation is successfully carried out a week later. It all sounds fair and reasonable. There are several aspects of this seemingly simple case that need careful scrutiny.

First of all, a patient never really needs a battery of diagnostic tests to diagnose any clinical condition and doctors should order a couple of tests at a time until they get there. But when money can be made by ordering more tests, whereas the alternative is delayed diagnosis and loss of patient confidence, very few doctors will actually follow sound scientific principles. Secondly, though you would like to believe that the ultrasound indeed showed gall stones, it is a presumption and may well be untrue. A friendly radiologist will not hesitate to write a few false words for his clinician friend in lieu of business sent. Finally, every surgeon knows (or should know) that, by and large, only patients with symptomatic gall stones need surgery. Gall stone is a common condition in any population and so are tummy pains. If you combine the two, you have a very common association between the gall stone and tummy pain. However, this association is not enough to recommend surgery. The surgeon or clinician needs to be reasonably confident that the patient's symptoms can be attributed to gall stones before recommending surgery. But when your survival is at stake and the alternative is a relatively easy operation, these scientific precautions seem unnecessary. Whether or not the patient needs this surgery is then a trivial obstacle, easily overcome. Whether or not the patient might suffer harm as a result of this unnecessary surgery becomes irrelevant.

No surgery is risk-free. We are talking about a procedure which, in the hands of even the best surgeons in the world, has a mortality (risk of dying) rate of approximately 1 in 500–1,000 and a major complication rate of 1–2 per cent. We are talking about an operation that can cost anywhere between Rs 50,000 and Rs 2,00,000. A common excuse one hears from doctors is that if they didn't do it, somebody else down the road will, and they are right. There is no shortage of new surgeons who will do anything to be able to earn a livelihood. Even if you are an established famous surgeon, you will only have the privileges of affiliation with a big corporate hospital if you can make money for them.

Moreover, you don't even need to be a surgeon to perform operations or, worse still, a patient could be admitted under a physician for an operation which is actually performed by a surgeon without the patient's knowledge. A number of 'ghost' surgeons are available for precisely such a situation. All that matters to these ghost surgeons is the money they make and the opportunity to be able to maintain their surgical skills. How can you perform an operation without explaining to the patient the risks involved, without ever even having spoken to the patient? These are some of the issues worth pondering over. But there's more to it. It is also an issue for society to collective think about. What other option do these fresh pass-out surgeons have, if they expect reasonably to live a decent professional life? Where can they work for good pay without having to worry about soliciting business? Yes, the system is somewhat flawed, but it would be naïve, and dare I say simplistic, to simply blame doctors for it. Lasting changes are only possible in human societies when all stakeholders accept their share of responsibility and work towards a change.

In the midst of all this, spare a thought for the poor patient who has now undergone a gallbladder surgery that she did not need. She is obviously lucky to have not had any complication (or death) as a result. She has possibly either taken the required money out of her savings or sold something to pay for the 'loot' that all the doctors and hospitals concerned, including her family doctor, the radiologist, the surgeon, the diagnostic centre and the hospital have shared. If she has an insurance policy, these bills will be borne by the insurance industry, and you perhaps know that the insurance industry doesn't really work for philanthropy either. So, as a direct result of such practices, insurance premiums would go up and everybody is a little bit worse off.

A similar, often-witnessed scenario involves patients with chest pain, cardiologists and insertion of coronary stents. Many professionals loosely use the term 'coronary stent syndrome' to refer to this phenomenon. Once again, the story is rather simple. A sixty-year-old man with chest pain goes to his local family doctor. His doctor suggests that it may be coming from his heart and that a cardiology opinion would be useful. The cardiologist then says that the patient may be suffering from coronary artery disease and an angiogram should help clarify the doubt and if it indeed shows coronary artery disease, it can be 'cured' by placing a stent. The patient duly undergoes a coronary angiogram. In the middle of the procedure, the cardiologist even calls another colleague for an independent second opinion. They concur and then come out to see the patient's family in the waiting area. The verdict is pronounced—the patient has serious heart disease involving two coronary vessels and needs stents. The patient's family could choose to not have it done but they will be going against medical advice and, of course, they will have to live with the guilt for the rest of their lives if the patient happens to have a fatal heart attack that very night. Moreover, the family members confer among themselves, what will he think when he finds out that his family refused this life-saving treatment? He will probably presume that his family put money above his life. Put this way, the choice is simple for any family. And they decide to go ahead with coronary stenting. The final bill can be anywhere between Rs 2 to 4 lakhs for two stents that cost the hospital Rs 60,000.

We will talk about the costs of appliances and drugs later. In this chapter, let us focus on whether the stenting itself was necessary. Chest pain is a common clinical condition and can result from a number of conditions. It promptly takes a patient to the doctor because deep inside, every patient is worried that it could be due to a heart problem. Family doctors and cardiologists are aware of this fear in patients' minds and will not hesitate to exploit it. If you carried out an angiography on everybody in any population, a lot of people will have some narrowing of their coronaries (the vessels that supply blood to the heart). But all of them don't need stenting as stenting has its own risks. There are very well-defined scientific criteria to help cardiologists decide where and when stenting is needed. However, as a doctor, when the survival of your own family is at stake and when the hospital has given you targets to achieve for the month, even the most conscientious cardiologist will not hesitate in recommending stenting even if it is not strictly necessary or required at all. Your friend (and you'd do the same for him) will be only too happy to confirm your management plan in the name of an independent second opinion.

I could go on and on and construct similar stories based on real life experiences of people I have spoken to or come across. A number of clinical conditions are especially vulnerable to abuse, but I will end this particular section by talking about the hysterectomy scandal. It was reported on BBC recently that there is a certain village in India where there is no woman left anymore with a uterus. Think about it. A forty-year-old lady has irregular periods. She goes to a gynaecologist following a recommendation by her doctor. The gynaecologist finds a uterine tumour on the ultrasound scan and recommends surgery. A hysterectomy (surgery to remove the uterus) is duly carried out. It all sounds perfectly genuine. What you may not know is that a very large number of women suffer with irregular or heavy periods. They don't all need surgery though. If you start scanning them all, a number of them will have completely benign (not cancerous) tumours in their uterus and a large number of these tumours won't need surgery either. Moreover, we mustn't underestimate what our friendly radiologists can write in their report in lieu of a steady stream of patients. *The fact that an ultrasound scan report says you have a tumour in your uterus doesn't necessarily mean that you have one.* Under these circumstances, it is perfectly possible that a lady with irregular periods, a condition that usually either eases on its own eventually or becomes manageable with some hormonal pills, ends up being diagnosed as a tumour and having a surgery.

In rural and semi-urban areas, many family doctors also dispense medicines and offer in-patient treatment in their clinics. In a market where a patient will willingly pay more when he comes home with some tablets to show for it or is given some intravenous fluid (commonly known as glucose drip), doctors have learnt to extract maximum money out of their clients. These doctors usually have one or two beds in their clinics and routinely treat patients with intravenous fluids, even antibiotics. Patients are supervised by a woman who is called the 'nurse' but has no professional qualifications really and the whole place is nothing more than a bed-and-drip-stand. How many of these patients really need one or two bottles of saline or glucose is anybody's guess but whatever little medicine I have come to understand, I know it is rare that any patient will ever need just one or two litres of intravenous fluids over a few hours and then become fit enough to go home.

Patients have no choice, especially when they are told that the alternative is admission to a hospital or nursing home, where the bill will usually run into lakhs. What patients probably don't know is that such practices don't decrease hospital admission rates. If you seriously do need in-patient hospital treatment, such practices usually mean that you are getting treatment in a facility that is not fit for the purpose and you will inevitably end up in a hospital anyway. Moreover, by the time you reach any hospital, your condition would have got worse, if not unsalvageable. If you didn't need hospital admission in the first place, which is usually the case when such treatment is administered in these clinics, you are wasting money on completely unnecessary, and potentially dangerous, treatment. When a doctor is dispensing medicines to you in paper packets and bottles, where is the sterility and quality control that we expect from the pharmaceutical industry? And how do you know what you are getting in the name of medicine? Indeed, many a times, these are simply placebos (sugar pills given in the guise of medicines in trials to examine effects of real drugs) being sold for a price.

Recently, a sting operation caught a physician in Delhi bribed into prescribing unnecessary nutritional supplements to a poor lady to meet a pharmaceutical company representative's targets. This again is a fairly common practice. If you go to a doctor and come back with a prescription for half a dozen tablets, you cannot presume that all of them have been prescribed to meet your health needs. As in this case, some of them may have been prescribed to keep medical representatives of drug companies happy.

Targets and Incentives

If you are the owner of a nursing home or a hospital, it is in your interest to keep the beds occupied and doctors working for you must know that it is their responsibility. Under these circumstances, it is not absolutely essential that a patient needs real in-patient treatment, as long as bills can be paid. On the other hand, if the patient cannot afford to pay the bills, it does not matter whether he will lose his life on the way to a government hospital, for he will not make it inside the private hospitals. One understands that private hospitals are not charities and they need to have a sustainable business model. But these businesses avail many government incentives and exemptions and it is only fair that the public gets reasonable returns on investment. I will attempt to specifically examine the private health care scenario later in this book.

You are sometimes deemed to need a bed for only as long as it takes to find somebody else to occupy it. Intensive and Critical Care beds are usually more expensive and once again admission criteria to these beds don't comprise purely clinical parameters. They are also determined by whether or not the patient can pay the charges and the targets that the doctor needs to meet. Though it is impossible to be certain of the extent of this 'target' culture, one hears about it from time to time. It is common knowledge that doctors working in many private establishments are given targets they must achieve to be able to keep their jobs. Even those hospitals that don't set a precise target monitor your activity.

Given our country's health care infrastructure, there is stiff competition among doctors for attachment with private hospitals. So these hospitals are in a position to determine the rules of the game. And the rule is actually pretty clear—you must be able to bring business to the hospital. This direct monetary reward system is one of the fundamental weaknesses of private health care systems in India. How can doctors be trusted to put the patient's interest first when it clashes every moment with their own? I would even argue that in any health care system, doctors should only be paid a wage—a decent wage commensurate to their social standing—and it must not be linked to whether they ask for more tests, admit more patients, or carry out more procedures. All health care systems, some even in developed countries, leave themselves open to abuse, when they incentivize doctors for individual activity.

It is my personal view that medicine can remain an honest and noble profession only if financial considerations can be removed from the day-to-day medical decision-making. Patients can implicitly trust their doctors only if they know that the doctor has only the welfare of the patient's health in mind, and no other vested interest. Patients will only be able to trust a doctor's advice if they know that the doctor does not stand to benefit financially from recommending the treatment or otherwise. Such is life. Sometimes, the presence of a motive is enough to make one a suspect, and this is nowhere more relevant than in the practice of medicine. Patients are in a desperate state when they seek medical advice and need to feel confident that the doctor will not take advantage of their vulnerability. If patients behave like shoppers and doctors like shop-owners, the medical profession cannot remain noble.

Doctors must provide circumstantially appropriate, scientifically sound, sympathetic and compassionate care, and in return, they should rightfully expect reasonable remuneration and some social standing. Sadly, the health care scenario does not play by these rules. Patients have little faith left in the doctors, as stories of unethical and sometimes, frankly unlawful behaviour, abound. A number of corrupt practices have gained hold over the medical profession, each more sinister than the other. And nothing rocks patient confidence in our medical establishment more than finding out that the tests and treatment recommended are sometimes intended solely for the purpose of squeezing money out of them.

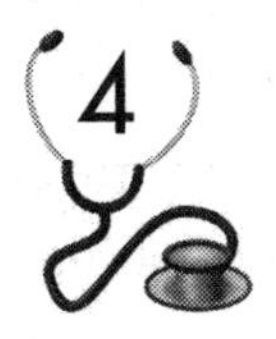

Drug Companies and Appliance Manufacturers

We didn't make this medicine for Indians...We made it for Western patients who can afford it.

—Marijn Dekkers, CEO of pharmaceutical giant Bayer

On sale of 1,000 samples of the drug, get a Motorola handset. On sale of 5,000 samples get an air cooler. On sale of 10,000 samples get a motor bike.

—Consumer International (quoting an Indian doctor)

It is impossible to talk about ethics in medical practice without discussing the relationship between corporates and doctors. Corporates can be multinational pharmaceutical companies, companies that manufacture medical appliances and instruments and, more recently in India, corporate hospitals. As is the case in the rest of the corporate world, the main objective in these establishments, too, is to generate profits for shareholders. And if they did this ethically, nobody in their right mind should or would question them.

It must be said that these corporates are absolutely vital to the practice of modern medicine and so it is important that the industry operates on a sustainable business model. For otherwise, who would invest the billions needed to develop a new drug, to see it through the stages of invention, development, trial, marketing and surveillance? Who would open new open hospitals in towns and cities across the country? And this is all the more important given the state of publicly funded hospitals. It is an undeniable fact that without corporate hospitals, millions of Indians will have nowhere to go for their health care needs.

Yet, it is also true that these corporate entities are largely responsible for erosion of traditional values and the advent of business culture in the world of medicine. For these organizations, running a hospital or manufacturing an appliance or selling a drug is business, it is a matter of survival in a highly competitive marketplace. But no matter how money-minded these organizations are, they can do little damage without the help of doctors—the custodians of society liaising between companies and patients.

Being well aware of this, companies develop marketing strategies aimed directly at doctors. They seek them out, make them feel important, shower them with expensive gifts, and if needed, even bribe them with cash to ensure continued sales of their products. The fact that many doctors are only too willing to participate in the process makes the job easier.

It has almost become a culture. It is now accepted practice for drug companies to periodically host lavish lunches and dinners for doctors in order to launch their products. It is also a fact that doctors can rely entirely on their own discretion to prescribe whichever brand they like. It is the norm that companies will sponsor meetings and conferences for doctors to travel around the globe and discuss important developments in lavish five-star settings. I am not saying that every doctor attending a major conference is being paid by a company, but it happens. Since these companies are not exactly charitable organizations working purely for human good, what do they seek in return?

What will persuade a company to send a doctor to a conference in Paris? Could this mean that the doctor will recommend its products even when a cheaper, better alternative exists? Does such selling of corporate goods to patients for a brokerage make a commission agent out of doctors? For if it does, it is a perfect brokerage business where the client, the patient, cannot question the agent, the doctor. Hospitals can be persuaded differently. Take, for example, two coronary stents—a commonly used medical device for patients with heart disease. Let us say these stents are of the same quality and bear the same displayed Maximum Retail Price (MRP) of Rs 80,000. One of these companies sells the stent to the hospital for Rs 70,000 (still leaving a good 15 per cent profit margin) and the other for Rs 35,000 (less than half of the MRP). Now can you guess which stent the hospital will ask its doctors to use? The same applies to pharmacies, when it comes to drugs. Companies are obviously free to price their drugs and devices the way they want. One does wish though that there was a regulatory body in the country to monitor these prices. Since both stents are approved, one can only presume that both are safe and effective. It is clear that the second company is passing on a huge amount of profit to the hospital (the retailer). The first company obviously doesn't want to go out of business. So what is it doing? Possibly, a number of things—the company may have higher costs (usually the case if the company manufactures outside India or has better infrastructure and other regulatory safeguards in place), or it may have a higher marketing/educational budget (usually includes sponsorship for conferences or for doctors to attend them) or it may simply be making more profit for itself rather than passing it on to the hospital.

It is a bit of a power game. Big corporates with significant leverage amongst the professionals are usually the first type; smaller local companies the second. In both cases, it is the patient who loses out and ends up paying much more for the treatment. This is hard-earned money that somebody saved at a few hundred every month or raised by selling some family assets or jewellery. These minor considerations, however, need not worry our hospitals or doctors as long as they have made some money or have had a paid holiday.

The Medical Leaders

Amongst doctors, some earn the tag of 'leaders' within the profession. They organize conferences and write guidelines. They set benchmarks and what they say becomes the clinical standard of practice. You disobey the diktats and leave yourself vulnerable to potential litigation from patients. The industry knows who these leaders are and they are carefully nurtured and pampered. They need lakhs of rupees to organize conferences in five-star hotels and ship in speakers from around the world in business class; the industry supports them. They need to travel around the world to retain their dominance; the industry funds it from the educational budget. It is all above board and done transparently. As long as you declare your competing interests, you can get away with endorsing or saying anything. Since these leaders are often also the editors of journals where researchers publish their findings, it is pretty difficult to develop any theory or ideas that oppose their views.

Companies know that ordinary doctors rely on published evidence to guide their practice. Now you might think of the world of science as pure and honest, where scientists develop concepts on the basis of hard evidence and the rest of the world uses this knowledge for patient care. The truth is slightly different. Research itself needs money, which is typically provided for by the government, charities and the industry. All of these providers want to see that you have some influence amongst your colleagues and peers before they trust you with their money. Now, since influence is an intangible asset that can be a bit difficult to measure, scientists use the number of articles they publish and the repute of the journals they are published in to gauge their own reputation.

That is where some of the biggest problems of the medical world lie. Journals where you can publish your research or ideas are a closely guarded club. You may wonder what is so difficult about this—you find something, you develop an idea and you share it with your colleagues. In this age of Internet, publishing and sharing ideas should be relatively easy. But that is not the case. For scientists to even be able to hear your ideas, you have to publish your findings in a journal which is indexed by major databases like PubMed, and preferably also indexed with the body that gives them what is called an impact factor. The impact factor ranks journals against each other and, depending on how many articles a scientist publishes in journals of high impact factor, it attempts to rank scientists too. It measures a journal and a scientist depending on how often their research is cited by others, and this citation is used as a surrogate marker of the impact of the journal.

Over the last few decades, this impact factor has become the most dominant mechanism for academicians and universities to assess each other. Its flaws are obvious. In sound language, it ranks scientists on the basis of the noise they create and not on the melody of their work. Scientists and journals dealing in contemporary, politically sensitive, popular and contentious issues are more likely to be cited. Whether or not they are correct or making any real difference, their impact will be higher. If you are a scientist working in a very narrow, niche field, you will need nothing short of a path-breaking invention to have a high impact factor. The problem is not to do with the impact factor per se; it is a tool with significant limitations that are widely acknowledged. The problem is with human psychology. Academics want to measure themselves against their peers and to this end, they will use whatever tool is available, even if it is a flawed indicator. It is like knowing that a massive Twitter following does not mean you are a good leader, yet a time will come when every worthwhile leader in the world will need to produce a sizable Twitter following to convince the rest of the world of his/her leadership status.

Journals that are indexed and have impact factors are run by big academics or societies, and owned by corporates. They only publish research or ideas that the editors and peers will approve of through a system referred to as 'editorial and peer review'. Fundamentally, this system places crowd approval over individual brilliance and this effectively means that though science will eventually move forward, it will only do so when all stakeholders are satisfied with the direction of progress. At every step, there are systematic influences. Coming to money or funding for research, you simply won't get any if you can't convince your peers or the gatekeepers sitting on the panels of these grants. Typically, these peers also look at your impact, which, as you now know, is measured on the basis of your publication in indexed journals. It is a closed club. Entry will require permission from people already in there and they will only let you in if you belong and won't rock the boat.

A lot of the research is conducted and funded by the industry. And it is a fact that industry-sponsored research more often tends to come out in support of their products and even if it doesn't (which happens less often), the industry is under no obligation to publish it. They can simply choose to not disclose the findings to anyone. So, if you think evidence-based science is honest science, documenting each step the human race takes into the world of the unknown and the hidden, think again. This document is a very selective portrayal of the journey; it only shows you what they want you to see. This document then forms the basis of clinical practice around the world—the day-to-day decisions that doctors make on your behalf.

Corporates know how this system works. They also know how to systematically benefit from it. They conduct trials; countries like India are becoming a popular place to host such trials because here it is easy to influence researchers and, should something go wrong, to suppress adverse publicity and legal damages. If the research they fund shows their product in poor light, they are simply not obliged to publish it. Any statistician knows that if you conduct enough number of studies, simply as a result of chance, some will incorrectly validate the wrong result. That is how statistics works; most of these studies will indeed show the right result to be statistically significant, but some will not. So, if you are only selectively going to publish findings and not publish all the studies conducted, you are, in effect, distorting scientific record. Statistics is an accurate science only if people are being honest. In the face of dishonesty and manipulative behaviour, statistics is powerless. So, these drug companies abuse statistics to further their aims. Trials showing their products in a favourable light are much more likely to be published and revealed to the wider medical community; the rest will fade away in history; and medical records will never reveal their existence.

Even if you are an independent researcher who somehow obtained money to carry out research and found something different, try publishing it in recognized journals. Many of the editors and the bodies that own these journals are not immune to the influence of corporates. Professional societies and associations need money to run. They need funds to organize their annual conferences and publish their monthly journals. It is difficult for these societies to take a view that harms the industry without losing the support the latter offers them. It's a very subtle drama and it's staged without a word exchanged; all the players know their part too well.

In reality, journals cannot keep an accurate record of all scientific activity. The scientific community treats journals a little bit like magazines. They should be interesting to read for doctors to want to subscribe to them. Journals publish what the readers enjoy and what will translate into improved journal subscription and citation (resulting in an increased impact factor). So, even if you wanted to publish all the negative findings, you'll struggle to find a journal that will do so. Though scientifically wrong, the reasoning behind this is easy to understand. Doctors don't want to be burdened with negative information about treatments and drugs that don't work. They want to read about things that do work, and that is why a trial reporting positive results is much easier to publish in reputed journals with high impact factors. Of course, this destroys the accuracy of scientific record by selectively recording only one type (positive) of results.

In today's times of unlimited digital publishing capacity, we have the opportunity and capability to publish every bit of scientific record that we want to and that will create an accurate chronological record of medical history. But there is another problem. Scientists who simply publish their thoughts or findings on platforms that are not indexed by the major bibliographic databases don't accrue any scientific merit for their work. Unless published in a journal which is tracked by these databases, work of even high quality is dismissed as a blog. You may wonder how science, which is supposed to be innovative by definition, could have a mechanism that needs the approval of peers in the field for you to be able to effectively voice your opinion. Even though it may sound counterintuitive, peer-reviewed publishing is currently the only respectable way to publish your scientific ideas. (My competing interest as co-founder and owner of a platform advocating post-publication peer review needs to be declared here.)

There is a system at work here—your academic success is largely dependent on what your peers think of you. Many of these peers have competing interests and have benefitted from the industry. I am not talking about overt bribing for prescribing a specific brand of medicine or even prescribing a medicine when a patient does not strictly need it, even though we have learnt from recent journalistic exposures that this goes on. I am taking about the industry systemically building opinion leaders and then using them for vested gains. Scientists have a mechanism for couching these competing interests. For example, if you have been paid by the industry for a lecture, you are supposed to declare it so that ordinary doctors and patients are aware that you may have another motive in promoting that drug or device. However, since almost all famous clinicians and researchers have significant competing interests, it is no more than lip service and does not really mean much at all. For example, journals do ask that you declare any competing interests, but there is no mechanism to police it if you didn't declare any significant ones, and even if you did declare them, it does not mean that journals will not publish your research. It simply means that readers will be informed of this in fine print at the end of the article. As a result, famous scientists get away with significant competing interests as it rarely has any influence on their day-to-day life and work.

There are also other well-established mechanisms in operation now for the industry to be able to influence opinions of key professionals. It is rare that professionals seek a direct bribe, although probably this happens as well. More commonly, they want to attend conferences in famous tourist destinations on a regular basis, sometimes with their families—all paid for by the industry of course. Many of them have no interest in presenting papers or even staying up-to-date with the latest. Some would skip whole sessions, even days, enjoying the touristic pleasures of conference cities. They don't even feel this is wrong. In fact, it has become a surrogate marker of your reputation. If a drug company is not sending you on a foreign holiday, you obviously don't have enough patients and are clearly not a famous doctor. It does not matter if you are simply unwilling to prescribe a much more expensive medicine when a cheaper alternative will do the job. It is truly a rat race and, unsurprisingly, the rats are winning.

Let us take a look at the conferences these doctors are attending. The underlying concept is fine. Researchers and doctors share their experiences and findings in a friendly atmosphere, bypassing the 'rigour' of academic journals and before the latest findings find their way into these journals. Such meetings are hosted by leaders of the profession on behalf of various local, national and international professional associations or societies. Though there is usually a fee for attending these meetings, costs are high and hosts can end up incurring losses if they don't plan carefully. Therefore, conference organizers depend on star speakers to attract delegates and many of these star speakers will only come if they are flown across the world in business class. All this costs money, which is partly provided by the industry. Within these conferences, there can be events sponsored solely by a company, with symposiums or lectures by their own star speakers. To be an industry-sponsored speaker, to be ferried around the world in business class for delivering lectures, you have to be on good terms with the companies and endorse their products. Many a times, leaders do this in the garb of evidence that they generate for the industry. Who can pose a challenge when a recognized leader of the profession tells you from a study he has conducted or from his own experience that a particular product or drug works better. They present studies that show the industry in flattering light. Those who don't indulge in such activities are less likely to get invited to big conferences as star speakers, either by the industry or the organizers, who themselves are dependent on the industry to share part of the costs of the event. On the other hand, if you are willing to work with the industry, you can even become a paid consultant, which effectively means you are on their pay roll for the services rendered. Put simply, it is payment for endorsement.

You are a famous doctor when you are teaching others. It does not really matter in this context if your own learning is far from complete and you could benefit from attending courses rather than hosting them. What matters is that you can provide business to the industry and suddenly the doors will open. Those clinicians in India, and perhaps in some other parts of the world, who have learnt to work with corporates are never short of such opportunities. The industry will help you earn the tag of an 'expert' by helping you organize these courses, even pay you to run them, and also by bringing new entrants in the field to you. In summary, if you are willing to teach others how to use their product, you can organize courses or have industry-sponsored fellows. All these go a long way towards establishing you as an expert in the field.

Building a Brand

If you are a surgeon looking to build your brand locally, you need to organize meetings for local doctors on a regular basis. You probably also need to invite patients to your 'support groups' to spread awareness of your brand. All this can be conveniently arranged by the marketing representative of the drug or appliance company you wish to support. Each of these measures will enhance your reputation amongst colleagues and patients. As you see, there is simply no end to what you can seek in return. The deal is very simple: you support them and they support you. The patient, whose money is ultimately at stake in all this, has no knowledge or say in these dealings.

Leaders of the profession need the umbrella cover offered by professional societies, the support of academic journals, and grants to retain their position. These work in synergy; you excel at one and the others will follow. Though it is possible for you to make a mark entirely independent of these, it will be very difficult. Moreover, most of your peers will have used one or more of these mechanisms and are widely respected by all. The end here justifies the means. If you do not follow these established pathways, you will be left behind.

This happens the world over, and companies don't even hide it. They have educational budgets to sponsor conferences where doctors and researchers interact with each other in lavish facilities over sumptuous meals. It's not all wrong either. Often, young doctors with limited study allowances get a chance to visit these conferences only because of generous funding from the corporates. The challenge for us as a society is to develop better mechanisms for sharing of scientific knowledge that can function without support from corporates.

Medical science has now progressed into the realms of invisible disease, and for good reasons. It is often too late by the time signs and symptoms of the disease are obvious. The outcomes of many diseases, a cancer for example, are very poor if the disease is not diagnosed early. Other conditions like high blood pressure and diabetes can go undetected for years. There is a genuine desire amongst medical professionals to improve public health by diagnosing and treating diseases at an early stage. This inevitably results in more visits to doctors and an ever-increasing number of diagnostic tests. For many conditions, there are even clearly laid out recommendations for screening normal populations. A direct consequence of this awareness is that even normal population is now within the ambit of the health care industry. One does not wish to challenge the screening of diseases in general but there is little doubt that many a times, screening tests are rolled out at mass population level without sufficient long term evidence. The world of clinical research where doctors collect and disseminate evidence to inform future patient care is far from perfect and not immune to human weaknesses. Doctors engaged in research often have significant conflicts of interest and benefit from promoting a specific drug, device or instrument. Moreover, they are often focussed on promoting their own narrow specialty or the interests of professionals working in it.

The Indian Reality

In India, the problem runs much deeper. Pharmaceutical and medical appliance companies here maintain an army of sales and marketing representatives, whose only job is to maintain a close relationship with doctors in every nook and corner of the country. The industry knows, of course, that availability of a good drug is not enough; you also need a willing doctor to prescribe it. It is the job of these medical representatives to convince doctors using logic and reasoning, and if that fails, with gifts or bribes. Small gifts like pens, medicine samples (as if medicine is a soap that the doctor has to use first before prescribing) and office accessories are all too common. But for a more willing doctor, the sky is the limit. Amongst doctors, there is some sort of competition. If one doctor is sent on a foreign conference trip to an Asian country, another wants to go to Europe. One got an iPhone, so another wants a laptop. Many doctors want cash, either legally as consultation fee or just plain cash in an envelope. An interesting state of affairs has come to exist, where gifts from the industry are an indirect measure of your reputation and popularity amongst patients and colleagues.

In return, companies ask for 'your support'. All you need to do is to prescribe their drugs or use their products, even if there is a much cheaper and better alternative out there. Whether or not your patient even needs this treatment is a small technicality, easily overcome. It should not matter that many of these patients can only afford the treatment by spending the kind of money it would take them weeks, months or even years to earn back. Similarly, manufacturers of hospital equipment, instruments and appliances, and the hospitals themselves, all benefit when you and I fall ill. There is a whole industry out there profiting from our illnesses. However, unlike other industries, where the manufacturers of goods can easily reach out to the final customers, this industry relies on an intermediary, the doctors. Without participation and help from doctors, this industry cannot function.

If a company is launching a new product or drug, or sometimes just to be able to retain their market share, they approach the 'leaders' among the doctors in the locality. Typically, these are either a consortium of local doctors, chapters of the Indian Medical Association operating in the area, or professional associations of speciality groups. Deals are struck. In return for lavish meals, companies get to advertise their products and also get speaker slots for a friendly clinician who is willing to openly support and endorse their product. Often, hospitals wishing to introduce new doctors to the local network of doctors also exploit the same route.

Drug Companies Regulator

Although things have taken a particularly ugly turn, the roots of this problem lie in the methods corporates around the world follow. It is no secret that many Western companies find Indian markets attractive. Given the relative stagnation in Western economies, the vast Indian market comprising a sixth of the world's population holds promise. In Western countries, the letter of the law is stronger and companies rarely cross a line. But in India, there is no effective regulator. And instead of helping to make things better, these multinational corporates have systematically used their resources to benefit from this culture. They blame their behaviour on the harsh realities of doing business in the country and then participate so effectively in market processes that the end result is a system far worse than the one they started out in. Although aberrations in ethical behaviour have existed in the Indian medical community for some time, it has become a systematized phenomenon over the last couple of decades and to a large extent, the blame lies with corporates manufacturing drugs and appliances as well as corporate hospitals. They have developed systems to allure doctors, who have, in turn, proved to be too weak in the face of temptation.

If there is a strong political will in place, the solution is rather simple. Companies could be forced to declare every paisa they spend on doctors, education and marketing in whatever form and aberrations can be punished severely. There simply is no legally binding code of conduct that applies to pharmaceutical companies at the moment. There are attempts by the Central Drug Standards Control Organization (CDSCO) through its Uniform Code of Pharmaceutical Marketing Practices and Organization of Pharmaceutical Producers of India (OPPI) to develop codes to regulate the industry, but these codes are voluntary, with no legal provisions. In a country where legal codes (such as that of the MCI for doctors) are routinely ignored, somehow I have little faith in a voluntary code. As we will see ahead in the book, CDSCO simply does not have the resources to monitor and implement a legally binding code, even if it had one. Moreover, in a country where every government-controlled body tends to attract controversy and corruption, perhaps we need to develop autonomous regulators with representation from a wide spectrum of society to aid the monitoring framework. I will attempt to discuss this in more detail later in the book.

Streamlining Continuing Medical Education

Continuing medical education is important. The medical field is evolving rapidly and doctors need to stay in touch with the latest developments. Medical conferences help achieve this. Moreover, organizing such events is a mark of leadership within the community. As a result, too many such five-star conferences and meetings are being organized around the globe at regular intervals, at huge costs. In case you're wondering who bears these costs, rest assured that they are ultimately borne by the patients and this only makes our health care more expensive. I think it should be possible for the scientific community to use digital technology more for the purposes of continuing education and to reduce the conference budgets. Of course, as a doctor, you should be able to spend time socially with peers and friends from all over the world in such comfortable hotels. All I am saying is that it should be at your own expense. To be honest, this is just one of those unfortunate things that the medical profession has gradually got sucked into. Individual doctors are doing it because everybody is organizing and attending these conferences. If we banned corporate contribution towards organization of such events, I am confident drug companies and the medical community will in due course discover equally good, if not better, mechanisms of sharing information and knowledge. Mechanisms can be established where companies can tell doctors about their new drug or devices without inviting them to fancy venues.

After all, educating doctors is not the responsibility of corporates and if you leave it to them, they will want something in return. In Chapter 3, we talked about Speciality Advisory Groups (perhaps under an Indian Institute of Clinical Excellence) to guide clinical practice. Later on in this book, I have argued for creation of a Postgraduate Training Focus Group for each speciality under a reformed MCI to oversee postgraduate education and training in their respective fields. I think for each speciality, the business of continuing medical education could then be delegated to these Postgraduate Training Focus Groups. These groups will do the job of furthering research within their respective areas, ensuring such research findings are shared with members on the ground using digital technology and developing virtual platforms for improved sharing and connectivity. The final experience may actually be better interaction and more connectivity than these conferences provide and at a lower cost. There is no doubt a certain number of medical conferences would still be required but they could be organized in medical colleges on a much smaller scale, and the video recordings shared with those who cannot attend to prevent them from degenerating into mega luxury entertainment shows. It will also mean that further investment will be required in building such fit-for-purpose facilities in our government medical institutions. The state of our government medical institutions and ways to revive them is a topic for another chapter.

One does not wish to be prescriptive. Numerous speciality associations across the country may still want to hold conferences for networking. As long as such events are funded entirely by the members, nobody could have any reasonable objection to them. In lieu, the members may be allowed tax exemption for such events. In my opinion, professional associations have two main functions. Firstly, they could provide representation to the speciality advisory groups and postgraduate training focus groups entrusted with the responsibility of developing guidelines and developing standards of training and continuing medical education respectively. Secondly, they could work as a lobby group, informing the government and the public on technical matters concerning their patients and members. Organization of an annual conference does not have to be their most important function.

Obviously, all these suggestions will call for a much wider debate within the medical profession. If the fraternity and the public feel that an annual conference is really necessary, it could even be part-funded by the government. One way or the other, we need to keep corporates away from the business of continuing medical education to prevent it from becoming a business.

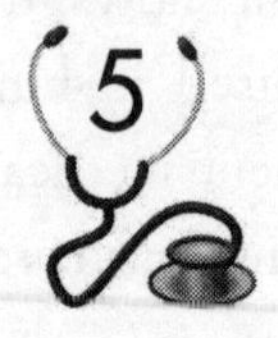

Exploitation of the Vulnerable and the Poor

Western pharmaceutical companies have seized on India over the past five years as a testing ground for drugs—making the most of a huge population and loose regulations which help dramatically cut research costs for lucrative products to be sold in the West. The relationship is so exploitative that some believe it represents a new colonialism.

—The *Independent*, 25 January 2015

Thousands of Indian women are having their wombs removed in operations that campaigners say are unnecessary and only performed to make money for unscrupulous private doctors.

—BBC News, 6 February 2013

Many Australians travel to India and pay surrogate mothers to bear their child. But the local women are often poor, desperate and exploited.

—The *Sunday Morning Herald*, 7 September 2012

Samastipur is one of the thirty-eight districts of Bihar. With a population of nearly three million, it has the unenviable distinction of being one of the most backward districts in the country. This sub-Himalayan landmass, boasting a rich culture of folk music and dance, has some very fertile plains irrigated by a number of rivers. The district borders the mighty Ganges to the South. Agriculture is the chief source of livelihood here; its lychees and mangoes are famous across the country. Like most of Bihar, Samastipur is plagued by low literacy and high crime rates. The social and political climate, associated with the high cost of acquiring fertile land for the purposes of industry, has meant that the benefits of industrialization have simply not reached these people. The fertile, sub-Himalayan plains blessed with abundant water—topographical features that must once have been huge assets—are no longer in demand. Lack of proximity to any big air/sea port or metropolitan city has meant that land prices have not seen the astronomical rise that places like Gurgaon have seen over the past couple of decades. Farmers here are largely poor and still believe that more male hands means more people who can work on the land. As a result, the region has one of the highest population growth rates and lowest sex ratios in India. Unlike most of the developed world, India's sex ratio is approximately 940 per 1,000 women, and for Samastipur, the number is an alarming 909. In 1992, Amartya Sen, Cambridge-based Nobel Laureate of Indian origin, described how social inequalities were skewing India's sex ratio despite the biological survival advantage that women seemed to have in other parts of the world. The shortfall in the number of women, which he referred to as 'missing women' with an academic detachment, has been variously estimated to be in excess of twenty-five million. Where are these missing women? This question will haunt a generation of Indian doctors, who you could argue were trusted to protect these unborn children, not abet their murders in the womb.

The Uterus Scandal

Sunita is considered lucky. She was allowed to be born, to grow up and marry a local boy from the same 'backward' community of Hindus. Her people have been subjected to systematic abuse for many millennia in the name of an Indian caste system, a not-so-glorious inheritance from our past that has prevailed for as long as you can trace back in the textbooks of history and mythology. Over the centuries, millions of such Hindus tried to take control of their destiny by even converting to other religions, only to realize that it will take more than a religion change to alter the bias deeply rooted in individual psyche and the collective social fabric. Architects of the Indian constitution tried to undo this age-old injustice by reserving places in educational establishments and government jobs for people from such socially backward background. Bold action was required to undo what was effectively an Indian version of slavery, and it has yielded results. We have seen massive benefits in terms of caste integration. Ambedkar changed with one stroke of a pen what we, as a society, had not been able to achieve in all our history thus far. People of upper castes were forced to change their opinion by the word of law. This proves what policy makers can do when popular opinion fails. It shows what leaders ought to do to nudge societies in the right direction. Politics, in democratic societies, has been reduced to an act of gauging public opinion and responding to it. Ambedkar was not a politician. He could take the risk of attempting to influence public opinion and not react to it. He did what he believed to be right, and his actions have yielded lasting results.

But even Ambedkar could not change Sunita's life. For Sunita, her husband, and her three kids, a small piece of land on the outskirts of one of the villages in Samastipur is their only means of earning a livelihood and a small 10-ft wide, 12-ft long and 6-ft high hut made of clay and tin roof, their home. This village has been home to their ancestors for generations together. They once had a big piece of land that spanned from the hill in the West to the canal in the East, but once divided among brothers (sisters were never involved in such sharing of family wealth) individual share of land was reduced to its current insignificant state over successive generations. Yet, this family is better off than many others. They can still live off their own land. They have seen many from the village move to cities like Delhi, Kolkata, Mumbai, Jaipur and Chandigarh in search of a livelihood. Most of these people work as house-help, waiters, labourers (on construction sites), rickshaw drivers, chauffeurs, or security guards.

For families like Sunita's, any illness poses a simple choice: selling all their assets or letting nature take its course. So, when the Government of India announced the Rashtriya Swasthya Bima Yojana (National Health Insurance Plan, if translated in English) in 2008 for people living below the poverty line, it was like help from the heavens. For Rs 30, they could get a card that would provide an annual hospitalization cover of up to Rs 30,000 for the entire family.

For several months, Sunita had been suffering from stomach (abdominal) pain and heavy periods. She had often thought of seeing a doctor. But the lack of a good female doctor in the village, busy family life, and worries about additional expenses made sure she kept putting it off. She knew that a visit to the doctor for the slightest of ailments was sufficient to derail the family budget for months. But lately, she was feeling more tired and the pain was getting more severe, until she could cope no longer. Moreover, this new government scheme meant that she would be able to have free treatment if it turned out to be something serious. And so it was that she finally went to see Dr Goyal.

Dr Goyal has been practising in Samastipur for nearly ten years. Over the years, he has built a large practice and a larger nursing home.

'How long has this been going on?' shouted Dr Goyal. There was always a big crowd in his clinic and he had to practically scream to be able to talk to his patients.

'Few months,' Sunita said in a whisper, still feeling awkward talking about her 'female' problems with a male doctor.

Dr Goyal asked a few more questions, carried out an examination and recommended an ultrasound scan and blood tests. Both tests were promptly carried out in his nursing home. It had cost Sunita Rs 700, an amount she had saved at Rs 200 a month by finely balancing the family finances. She had known Dr Goyal would ask to get tests done; he always did, but he was a good doctor. People like Sunita are naïve; they presume that doctors can only become rich and famous if they are good. What they have no way of knowing is that the methods that make doctors rich and famous are usually different from those that make them good.

'You've got cancer of the womb and you need an operation today to remove it,' said Dr Goyal with a hint of compassion in his voice and almost absolute authority. He had learnt over the years that he could not leave any doubt in patients' minds as that inevitably resulted in them seeking a second opinion and not coming back.

'Fine, Doctor Saheb, I will speak to my husband and let you know in a day or two,' Shanti said in her rural dialect.

'You don't get it,' said Dr Goyal politely, 'the tumour can burst anytime and kill you. You are lucky; I have some time today. You can see how busy I am.'

'How long will the operation take, Doctor Saheb? Are there any risks? I have two little children. How much will it cost? How long will I have to be in the hospital?' All the questions surging in Sunita's mind came tumbling out in one breath as she sensed that the good doctor was getting impatient and that if she didn't decide quickly, she may be putting her life at risk.

'You have a smart card, don't you? (People who subscribed to the government scheme were given a smart card.) For you it is free. The government will pay for it. It is a small operation and there is no risk. I will send you home tomorrow.'

Sunita was relieved and proud at the same time. She had come to Dr Goyal at the right time. If she had delayed any longer, what would have become of her kids? She agreed to go under the knife. The surgery was safely carried out and she was indeed sent home the morning after. She is and will forever remain grateful to Dr Goyal for saving her life. After all, she will never find out the truth.

What you just read is a fictional story built around some newspaper reports. What follows is not a figment of imagination though. Samastipur's District Magistrate Kundan Kumar was chairing a meeting to ensure successful implementation of this ambitious health insurance scheme launched by the Manmohan Singh government in his local area. A large number of payments were being made for this operation called 'hysterectomy'.

Hysterectomy is Latin for removal of the uterus or womb. Out of a total of 14,851 procedures conducted under this scheme between 2010 and 2012 in sixteen hospitals listed on the panel, a startling 5, 503 were hysterectomies. In some hospitals, this operation accounted for more than half of all the operations performed. Kundan Kumar then started examining tariffs for individual operations. This operation had one of the highest tariffs. He suspected a medical fraud. Why was it that so many of one single type of surgery were needed in his area? Were some doctors systematically manipulating the scheme? He had to dig deeper.

Mr Sharma organized an elaborate five-day medical camp and invited women who had undergone a hysterectomy under this scheme in Samastipur. A total of 2, 600 women attended the camp and were examined by an expert panel of doctors. The findings of the panel provoked a national and international outrage. The panel concluded that 717 patients had unwanted surgery; 124 underwent under-age surgery; there were 320 cases of fleecing and 23 cases of non-surgery. If you are struggling to understand what non-surgery means; it implies that the patient was taken to an operation theatre, put to sleep, her abdomen was opened up with a surgical knife, just as you would do with a standard hysterectomy operation, but the surgery was never carried out and the patient was simply stitched back. No wonder, these patients then made a swift recovery as they never really underwent a hysterectomy!

Soon, such reports started pouring in from other districts of Bihar and from other parts of the country. This was truly turning out to be a pan India phenomenon. Samastipur was the tip of the iceberg and merely a symptom of a much deeper evil lurking in

Indian health care. As if to prove this point, then president of the Bihar chapter of Indian Medical Association, Dr A.K. Thakur was reported to have challenged the findings of this expert panel and denied the existence of any racket. In any democratic institution, office-bearers must represent the majority view to get elected. But for societies to move forward, once a leader is elected, he must do what is right and not just what is popular. Sadly, these can be two very different things. Many elected leaders with their eyes on re-election often forget this and continued pursuit of power makes it a difficult principle for them to follow. Dr Thakur was no exception.

The insurance scheme that was supposed to protect the health of these poor people became the very vehicle of their exploitation. Since hospitalization was mandatory under the scheme, these patients ended up being unnecessarily hospitalized and operated upon. Insurance fraud happens in other countries too, but a situation where completely unnecessary operations could be carried out on such a large scale is probably unique to India. There can be obvious questions raised about various professional associations, medical regulators, government bodies, law machinery, and so on, but none of this will answer how a doctor could exploit the poor in society in this mercenary manner.

When it comes to treating the underprivileged, the track record of humanity in almost all parts of the world is nothing to be proud of. It was only in 1834 that the British Slavery Abolition Act came into force and wiped out the disgrace of slavery throughout the British Empire. In the 1980s, when I was growing up in Kolkata, it was commonplace for us children to be asked to take a shower if we inadvertently touched a 'bhangi'. Bhangi was the term used to denote very poor men or women who came to clean our toilets, who almost universally belonged to the lower castes in society. They would have to be content with the food and clothes that we were ready to discard. Since we ourselves weren't very well off, it only meant that the leftovers passed on to these people were often not suitable for human consumption.

Doctors come from the same society as the rest of us and carry the same beliefs and prejudices. If medical corruption is an isolated phenomenon in the Indian set up, it will then have to be examined as such but if it is just one of the symptoms of a systematic decline in values affecting all of society, we will have to look elsewhere for solutions.

The Willing Organ Donor

If you think the state of Indian health care is broken, too expensive, exploitative and difficult to navigate, spare a thought for those living below the poverty line. It is as if all the developments of the human race have simply passed them by! How human life survives in all its glory in such abject sub-human conditions is beyond my comprehension. I will not pretend to understand what it must feel like to look for food in the stinking heap of garbage by the wayside that most people can't get past without holding their breath. Nor would I ever know how it feels when someone's children are begging with them on the streets. Do we ever think about the families of labourers who built our apartments and houses with their bare hands? How do they survive on their meagre earnings day after day, night after night? How hope survives in such a hopeless environment is one of the most perplexing mysteries of our times.

Salim came to work in Gurgaon five years ago from a little known village in eastern Uttar Pradesh. Uttar Pradesh and Bihar are probably two of the most underdeveloped states in India, and you can see people like Salim in almost all major cities. It is particularly difficult for poor Muslims in India, as most Hindus, who largely control the economy and the administration, prefer to hire people of their own faith. Despite centuries of sharing the same streets and neighbourhoods, there is a trust deficit in the Hindu–Muslim relationship. Partition on religious grounds in 1947 did not help and with little knowledge of all the political manoeuvring that saw India become a secular state, Hindus in India cannot forget that while Muslims got Pakistan and Bangladesh, they got no 'Hindu' state. A certain section of Indian Hindu population (which seems to be growing rapidly) feels hard done by.

There are other forces at play. At a time when practitioners of Islam often put their religious identity before other identities, Indian Hindus are not the only ones questioning their loyalty. In the current world order, national identity has emerged as the strongest form of identity, and its betrayal in favour of other identities attracts universal disapproval. Whether we really want to arrange identities in some sort of a pecking order or alternatively focus on teaching people to be tolerant and empathetic towards others with a broader sense of identity are choices that almost all societies across the world face today. India is no exception.

The livelihood of Salim, his two younger brothers and parents back home depended on Salim's cycle rickshaw. Salim had been through many a job 'interview' in the past, but none had ever progressed beyond his name. Riding a cycle rickshaw was easy, as nobody was really interested in your name. Often, he would give a Hindu name when asked. Working twelve hours a day, riding his rickshaw from one place to another for sums of Rs 20, Rs 30, Rs 40, Salim would earn about Rs 500 in a day. He earned much less over the weekend and on the holidays. But he was much better off as a result of coming to Gurgaon. In the village, there was no food, no work and nowhere to live for the growing family. His parents could barely feed themselves, but that had not prevented them from bearing eight children.

Salim had rented a small room in Gurgaon for Rs 3, 000 per month. He lived there with his wife, three-year-old daughter, and two younger brothers who had come over from the village to follow in his footsteps. He would need to buy two more rickshaws. Salim needed Rs 15,000.

'Do you want a job?' the stranger asked Salim near the teashop. Salim did not know him but he had seen this man talking to others in this narrow street in the old town section of Gurgaon. 'Doctor Saheb is looking for a good assistant who can speak Urdu. He gets lots of patients from Pakistan. Interview is tomorrow morning. Get here before 10 a.m.,' so saying, he handed a slip to Salim.

Salim was on time. He was surprised to see gunmen in the waiting room and assumed that the doctor was a famous man who saw patients from all over the world. Surely he had to protect them. Then somebody came up from behind, pinned Salim to the ground and put a gun to his head. Before he could get a sense of what was happening, he had been injected with something and fell unconscious.

He woke up in a hospital bed. There was a dressing to the left of his abdomen where it hurt a bit. Then the same man who had met him at the tea stall came up to him and said, 'Your kidney has been removed. Take this. There is one lakh rupees in this packet. It is much better than the market price. Doctor Saheb pays a good rate to everybody.' Salim was too confused to think and simply wanted to get out of this place.

World over, there is a shortage in the availability of human organs required for transplants, but in Western countries, a majority of the supply comes from dead or dying (brain dead) individuals. It is a fact that many patients who need organs die on the transplant waiting lists. In India, given the lack of faith in doctors (who, some patients worry, might just declare you dead so as to procure your organs) and cultural issues, cadaveric organ donation is almost non-existent. At the same time, an abundance of the desperate poor means that there is no shortage of potential living organ donors. Match the two and a perfect market is born. In this market, the poor can sell their organs to keep the rich alive as if just to prove the point that if societies allow everything to be traded, we will truly stop at nothing. People argue for organ trade to be legalized, but then there are people who also argue for prostitution to be legalized. Now, I am no expert on poverty control nor do I know what feels worse—to have no food or to live as a prostitute, to watch your kids go to sleep hungry or to live with one kidney. What I do know is that the solution to poverty problems is not organ trade or prostitution; it is control of population growth and fair distribution of wealth and resources. Besides, if we were to legalize these things today, what are we going to legalize next?

The fact remains that prohibition of organ trade has not prevented exploitation of the poor for organs. It has actually led to the creation of a whole new system where touts can arrange donors and also coach them to cheat the 'willing' transplant ethics committees. Many touts even operate in collusion with committee members, medical teams and hospitals. And laws often end up victimizing those they were meant to protect.

Poor Surrogate Mother

There is something about birth and death that can lead even an ordinary human being down the path of philosophical meanderings. If living in the here and now is a practical reality, thinking about the before and after is a profound human spiritual need. Delving into the unknown and the beyond is an eternal human quest that can never end, for if it did, life, as we know it today, will also end. Fear of that unknown higher form of justice acts as a monitor of human behaviour and in lawless societies such as ours, it is perhaps the only real regulatory force. Many have hence argued that medicine should not be allowed to interfere too much with the building blocks of life. The core purpose of medicine is to facilitate safe and healthy birth, a good life and a peaceful death, whilst ensuring that life is not prematurely cut short.

One cannot argue against the merits of individual scientific advancement but we need a sufficient lag period before radical medical advancements are allowed to become routine practice. We live in an age where advancements and inventions are being incorporated in our life at breakneck speed without enough safeguards in place. Often, the true impact of these developments is not clear until several decades later, by when of course the members of the scientific panel who approved incorporation of these developments are either retired or dead.

Over the last ten years, three-parent babies have become a reality where babies are created in designer style out of not just the mother's and father's genetic material but with a third woman contributing the mitochondrial DNA. In a nutshell, it means the child is born with genetic material from two women and one man. Scientific advancements have broken down the process of birth into multiple steps that operate independently of each other. It is only a matter of time before we will see four or even more parents involved in creating a baby. Imagine a scenario where sperm from a man, nuclear DNA from a woman and mitochondrial DNA from another woman create a human embryo, which can then be implanted in a third woman to actually 'bear' the child and give birth. Which of the three women will be the child's mother? There is little doubt that such developments allow women afflicted with diseases transmitted through mitochondrial DNA to have 'normal' children. Nonetheless, it represents an interference with some very basic human processes that we don't yet fully understand. The ability to break down the individual steps involved to replicate a biological process cannot be equated with understanding it. Those among us who are adventurous or after academic recognition and professorships will always be able to seek and find justification to push boundaries. In modern times, such academicians with unlimited ambition pose greater danger to mankind than aliens or armies of robots. Knowledge is an ally but it needs wisdom to guide it.

Surrogate motherhood is a similar development that uses our ability to break down these natural processes of birth to help some women have children of their own. It allows couples to use a third woman's uterus to implant and carry the child until it is born. I don't know, probably never will, how a woman feels when the child she has carried for nine months is separated from her soon after birth. Does she feel less of a mother because of the technicalities involved? Does she feel she sold her child for money? Will this child ever want to know who nourished and nurtured him/her for those nine months? Poverty, though, makes you do radical things. There are plenty of such women in India who will do anything for money and it should hardly surprise you to learn that India is emerging as a major centre for surrogate motherhood. After all, it is a legal business here. It does not matter if these women cannot read or understand the consent forms, don't know the risks to their health, and often end up paying a significant share of their income to the middlemen, who are usually hired by the doctors themselves.

When the choice is between having nowhere to live and seeing your children starve on one hand and an option that can take care of both these basic human needs, decision-making becomes easy and doubts disappear. These are the fundamental dynamics driving India's surrogacy industry. It is estimated that nearly 20,000 such pregnancies have taken place in India over the last decade. Women renting out their wombs to wealthy Western couples are typically poor and in a desperate state. They are paid between two to three lakh rupees for their services. In return, they forfeit any right to call the child their own, have to live in a 'secure' environment (where they can only meet their relatives once a week), and of course, take the risk to their health and life that comes with pregnancy.

Left to the discretion of market forces, we know human character knows no scruples. So civilized societies expect elected representatives to establish mechanisms to keep these market forces in check. A number of these surrogacy clinics have come up in India because it is good business. They can charge their Western customers five to ten times the money they pay these women. At an approximate charge of USD 25,000 per pregnancy, the industry is worth a meagre USD 30 million to the Indian economy—hardly a sum of money that should encourage one of the top ten economies in the world to leave its poorest exposed to exploitation by rich Westerners who couldn't care less about these women as they are 'paying' for the services. There is a reason why 'commercial' surrogacy is banned in most of Europe. It has to be the wider responsibility of the state to lay down clear rules on what can be sold and bought in a society and to set a fair price for it.

'The vulnerability of poverty is being exploited in this whole system. It should be banned. It should not be allowed,' Ranjana Kumari, a noted woman's rights activist, has been quoted as saying. Dr Kumari is right. Apart from all the emotional upheaval that these women must go through, they also risk complications of pregnancy and in worst-case scenarios, death. It is not too hard to anticipate who the doctors will want to save if they have to choose between the life of the mother or the child if things go south. And if the woman develops any late pregnancy related complication, she may even end up paying for it from her own pocket. By then, the new parents and the child would be back in their safe and comfortable homes in Europe or Australia.

An Australian couple recently went through this process in Thailand. A pair of twins—a boy and a girl—were born. This case, however, led to international outrage and Thailand banned surrogacy after the couple fled the country with the healthy girl child, leaving behind the boy born with Down's Syndrome. Down's Syndrome children often suffer with learning disability but can otherwise live a normal life. Yet, these 'parents' abandoned the boy. In my view, this happened because they were shopping for goods and clearly didn't want to accept 'sub-standard' products they thought they had paid full price for. They simply had no connection with the baby who was left for the surrogate 'mother' to look after. Similar instances have been reported elsewhere, including India.

Anand is a city on the western fringes of the country in the state of Gujarat, connected with other major cities of this prosperous state with good road and rail links. Most native Gujaratis are relatively well off by Indian standards thanks to thriving agriculture, dairy farming and industry. Anand, like the rest of Gujarat, is an example of the success of Gujarati entrepreneurship. But there is no shortage of people with little or no means in the villages around the city and amongst those who have migrated here in search of a livelihood from other parts of India. This scenario provides a rich supply of poor labourers, essential for local industry. It is in the interest of industry to maintain a 'healthy' competition among labourers. We have a number of mechanisms to ensure 'fair' competition among industries but there is none to protect the poorest in the society. There is a prescribed minimum wage laid out by law but, truth be told, it is not universally implemented.

If we looked around us, we would find innumerable victims of uncontrolled capitalism, where the rich accumulate an obscene amount of wealth with complete disregard for the people who make it possible for them to do so.

Sonal, one such victim of unchecked capitalism, lives in Anand. She lives in a slum, in what can only be described as an enclosure guarded by brick. The walls are roofed with a combination of plastic sheets and tin, held in place by bricks and stones. Thankfully, it doesn't rain much in Anand; for the flimsy roof leaked and the place got flooded when it did happen. This is home for Sonal where she lives with her husband and two children. Her husband earns Rs 4, 000 a month as a vegetable vendor. It must be a cruel joke of fate that his family can't afford to eat the vegetables he sells from morning till late afternoon. In the evenings, he works in a local restaurant for an additional Rs 2, 000. Life isn't exactly easy for them, but it is better than the one they left behind in the village they came from, where there was no work and no food. Here, they are happy and thank God often. Such is this world—people given the least are often the most thankful. It must be one of nature's ways of ensuring fair play that happiness does not depend on material possessions. The poor in society sometimes believe that wealth will bring them more happiness. The rich find out it that it does not, but hypothesize that it must be the relative lack of it and go out seeking more.

Sonal knew that life was hard for her husband. He walked through half the city all day and then worked again till late night. This was his daily routine every day of the week, month and year. When he couldn't go out, he didn't earn anything, and that meant he rarely took a day off. Sonal wanted to help but there was little she could do.

One day, Roshni, her neighbour, was moving out as they had bought a new house.

'Come and see us sometime,' Roshni invited Sonal to her new home with both a sense of pride and affection.

'We will,' Sonal said, her eyes welling up as she held Roshni in a tight embrace. She was sad to see her go. Roshni and Sonal had become such close friends. They had no secrets from each other.

'Think about what I said. There are no risks and they really take care of you,' Roshni said, as she was leaving. Roshni had told Sonal about this clinic where a woman could earn a lot of money for simply carrying a child for a 'foreign' couple.

'You must be out of your mind. Mother and father will never accept it,' Sonal's husband had reacted angrily when she first mentioned the idea to him.

'Think how much they are paying. We can never save that much all our lives. I will be able to send our children to the school,' she tried to convince him.

But he wasn't prepared to listen. 'What if my parents find out? This will certainly ruin their reputation in the village—my wife carrying somebody else's child!'

'How will they? We will visit them before I go to the clinic and we never visit them twice in a year anyway. Besides, Roshni has promised to look after our children. I have thought about everything.'

It took many emotionally fraught nights of pleading and persuasion before Sonal's husband agreed to the idea, but only on the condition that his parents should not find out about it under any circumstances. He did not want to bring any shame upon his family.

Sonal signed up with the clinic right away. She went through the medical check-up and a training programme where she was told everything about the whole process. A month later, she met this couple from Europe whose child she was to conceive. The woman had been left incapable of carrying a child after an operation on her womb. They seemed desperate for offspring. They were good people. Sonal was helping them. She suddenly felt very good about what she was doing. After the first five months, she lived in the clinic where she shared a dormitory with ten other women. They were all given good healthy food and bedding and clothes that were very comfortable and clean by her standards. She made many good friends there. Her own children at home were told their mother was ill and in a hospital. They all came to see her every Sunday.

She gave birth to a boy whom she was not allowed to even hold in her arms once. As soon as the child was born, he was whisked away to his biological parents who were waiting for his arrival. Sonal cried and cried. She had wanted to hold 'her' child and feed him, but any deepening of an emotional connection can cause future problems. Dr Gupta, who ran the clinic, had a strict policy that women should not have any contact with these children after birth. It was a purely commercial contract. Dr Gupta was convinced she was providing a valuable service to both the women involved. In this world driven by business, everything has a price tag, including the bond between a mother and a child. Sonal is lucky. She is alive, suffered no complication, the boy she gave birth to is healthy, and since there was no middleman involved, she will get the full amount of money promised.

As she left the clinic, Sonal tried hard to hold back her tears, thinking of her 'other' children at home. She knew she had no choice. Surrogacy had lifted them out of abject poverty. The city seemed to swarm in its usual frenetic rhythm all around her. Everybody was busy minding their own business. Nobody had the time or inclination to ask Sonal why she was crying. Were they tears of joy or sorrow? Nobody, not even Sonal, knows the answer to this question.

The Guinea Pig

In this market-obsessed world, an abundance of any product drives its price down, and that is the story of everyday human life as well. Whoever can exploit the poor will exploit them. The mighty pharmaceutical giants too have spotted a huge surplus of (cheap) human life in India. Regulatory agencies the world over want to see human trials before approving any drug and we all know human studies are not easy to conduct. There are a number of guidelines that must be followed to ensure such trials are conducted on well-informed participants who understand the risks and benefits. When the industry knows that this is a country where multinationals can kill many thousands and get away with it (simply compare the British Petroleum accident in USA in 2010 to the Bhopal gas tragedy and you'll understand what I mean), they are not going to worry too much about all the appropriate safeguards needed. Moreover, they don't even have to be directly involved. They can outsource trials to Indian companies who will do everything for them including recruiting patients, conducting the study, and massaging the figures if need be. Basic safety precautions are often ignored; doctors are bribed to recruit patients; the process of acquiring consent can be rudimentary or non-existent; and data, well, God only knows how accurate that is. At the end of it all, we get drugs that are so overpriced that they remain out of reach of the people they were tried upon. The grand justification given by the industry: 'We don't make these drugs for Indians. We make them for people in Western countries who can afford them.'

There is a new trend we are seeing in medical conferences—of live operating on patients. The idea is simple. Expert surgeons perform live operations in front of delegates sitting in a conference hall. Though one can see how such activities can add to the entertainment value and learning experience of a medical conference, I am not sure the art of learning surgery needs to be lowered to this level. Which patient in his right mind, when informed of all the details clearly, will agree to be operated on for an audience? When such conferences are organized by government hospitals, patients are typically poor with little say in the matter, and when it comes to private sector hospitals, patients are lured with massive discounts.

We are talking about real surgery on real human beings. We are talking about operations that can be dangerous, even without the additional stress that the surgeon must feel when being watched by hundreds of peers and colleagues. Patients can die as a result of 'live conference operating' just like patients can die during any surgery. The real issue here is whether we as a society or group of professionals want to turn the art of learning surgery into a road show. Can the same benefits be derived from watching the videos of operations in your bedroom? Yes, it is possible that the surgeons may not want to share embarrassing moments freely and videos may not be accurate representations of the reality but I would argue that operating in front of a crowd is not a real life scenario either. Are accidents more likely to happen when you are performing in front of hundreds of people? Are you going to be able to deal with any complication that may arise during the operation as effectively as you otherwise would? I don't think so. In any case, if conference organizers must do it, they must ensure that there is a board comprising 'accountable' professionals overseeing the whole process who then shoulder the ultimate responsibility for such actions and also intervene as and when necessary. To leave all the decision-making to the operating surgeon, who is not only under enormous pressure but also trying to protect his reputation, is not fair on the unsuspecting, usually ill-informed, patients.

Once upon a time, surgeons regarded operating theatres as temples; now, they behave like live chat show hosts. The transformation is taking place right in front of our eyes.

The Vulnerable

A patient is in a vulnerable, agitated state and a doctor is in a powerful position of trust. It is up to the doctors how to use this privilege—to heal the sick or to exploit them. You can either use a patient's fear of disease or suffering to make more money, or use your position to calm the patient. How desensitized must one become to extort somebody's life savings by performing an unnecessary operation, or to sexually exploit somebody trusting you with everything, or to rob the poorest in the society to meet the targets of multinational pharmaceutical giants. The rich and the educated are not easy to fool. They can look after themselves.

What about an uneducated, young, poor woman who trusts her doctor with all she has?

Social Evils

Doctors are men of science who use the latest in scientific development to prevent, control or cure diseases. However, in wrong hands, this knowledge can prove dangerous. It is commonly known that in the recent past, abortion of female foetuses has gone on a mass scale in India and, even now, when the regulations are much tougher, it continues to happen. This has skewed the sex ratio of an entire society.

It is also common knowledge that many doctors carry out illegal abortions outside the approved guidelines. Girls with subnormal mental function are at risk of getting sexually abused by members of the family and others. Doctors can help you there by carrying out a hysterectomy (surgery to remove the womb or uterus) so these women will never fall pregnant and the sexual predators can do what they like. Doctors in many countries are under pressure to perpetuate social evils. Female genital manipulation seen in many countries is one such example. But doctors take an oath to protect the vulnerable, to not harm the most vulnerable in the society on the pretext of social custom. Though, when the choice is between losing business by standing up for the right or making money by indulging popular beliefs, the decision is easy.

No Easy Way Out

As you will see, each chapter in this book attempts to make suggestions for the future, in exploring how we can change things, as I firmly believe that simply reiterating the problems will not do justice to what we have set out to achieve with this book. But in this chapter, I am at a complete loss. How do you instil values in people? How do you teach people to be sympathetic? How do you teach social equity and fair play? How do you teach humans to be humane?

The more I think about these issues, the more my mind turns towards our education system—both in the early formative years and subsequently in medical colleges and university. It is my impression that our education system focuses too much on collecting and imparting information and too little on thinking, analysing and understanding it. Teachers and parents need to think about how to raise children who are going to become responsible citizens—men and women who can place the collective good above individual benefit. The education system must fight against the dehumanization of those living in extreme poverty. Children need to be taught to see those in dire poverty as fellow beings. They need to understand what the poor go through and they must know that it is our shared responsibility to ensure everybody has a decent quality of life. In medical colleges, there should be open discussions and debates on social values and ethics. Currently, the medical curriculum concentrates almost entirely on the science with little emphasis on the social aspects, morality and ethics involved. Instead of doctors, we are producing armies of medical robots removed from the society they work in.

Poverty is the biggest curse in human society and yet, all the advances of the human race have only helped increase the numbers of those living out the cruel realities of poverty. It is a fact that the poor suffer most from the corruption or failure of law and order. It is not enough for the government to redefine the poverty line to make statistics look better. Successive Indian governments have failed to ensure that everybody in the country can earn a respectable living wage. Government schemes designed to help the poor have made them more vulnerable to abuse and exploitation. None of this will be easy to change. Can it ever change?

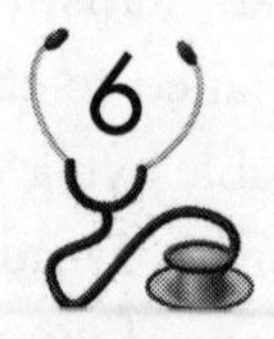

The Touts

The touts can get your tests done quickly for a fee, get you a bed despite the hospital staff telling you that all are occupied, fix up appointments with doctors for a charge, help you get medicines by overcharging, and even provide blood bottles in a jiffy.

—*Hindustan Times*, Ranchi, 13 June 2015

With their vast network among hospital staff, the touts can get your tests done in a day, get you a bed despite the authorities telling you that all are occupied, help you navigate the complex buildings, and make sure your stay in the hospital is comfortable.

—Mail Online, India, 25 Jan 2015

They offer 'help' in getting an appointment, and have records examined and signed by the doctors. Many touts have acquaintance with doctors and knowledge of the functioning of the hospital. People in the country pay Rs 2,017 crore a year as bribes in government hospitals.

—Divya Ramamurthi and Raghava M., The *Hindu*, 31 May 2006

The Medical Council of India warns doctors explicitly: 'A physician shall not use touts or agents for procuring patients.'

Medicine has become a business, and one sure way this reality manifests is in the way the art is reduced to a commodity that must be sold. In the unregulated, unsupported environment that private doctors work in in this country, attracting patients takes up a major part of their time and effort; the kind of time and effort that one hopes would otherwise be spent looking after patients and developing science. No surprise then that our doctors generally do very poorly in pushing new frontiers and the contribution of Indian private sector doctors to global scientific media literature is miniscule.

Touts constitute one of the most interesting aspects of health care in India. It may even sound funny if it did not have really serious consequences. You've got these helping hands all over the place. They act as middlemen and appear from nowhere, precisely when you need such help. They have contacts in high places. Depending on your need, they can arrange anything and everything. They will get you to the right doctor, the right laboratory and the right hospital, just when you are beginning to feel lost in a new city. In lieu, they will take a commission either from you or from the doctor or laboratory or hospital, depending on the services provided. For example, touts from villages will barge into doctors' offices in towns and cities, declare to the doctor that they have 'brought' a patient, explain what they want the doctor to do, clarify how deep the patient's pockets are, and finally agree on the commission with the doctor. Depending on how desperate the doctor is, the commission can be quite substantial.

This phenomenon is by no means specific to rural patients seeking help in big cities. In urban practice, it takes different forms and is rampant in both public and private sector hospitals. In the public sector, these touts are sometimes the channels whereby government doctors and officers earn extra money. In the private sector, they are employed by many doctors, laboratories and hospitals to attract patients. They prey upon the sick at a time when they are most vulnerable, masquerading as God's angels. These are a thriving community unto themselves—the Indian medical touts.

In a very poor country like ours, there is no shortage of people who will do anything for you for any wage. For a monthly salary in the range of Rs 10,000 to Rs 20,000, you can hire any number of 'marketing executives' or 'secretaries' or 'personal assistants' you like. In a market where one can make tens of thousands of rupees from just one patient, many hospitals and nursing home owners know that such employees finance their own employment and it pays back to have as many of them around as possible. The job is simple—they have to ensure a constant stream of patients. This means interacting with local doctors and establishing deals. This also means tying up with quacks and RMPs in villages. We have dealt with this world of cuts and commissions in an earlier chapter. There is a third method of getting patients to a clinic or a hospital—via a tout who preys upon helpless patients in government hospitals, at bus stands, railways stations, or anywhere else. Obviously when one gets better at this job, one won't work for Rs 10,000 a month, and voila! A freelance tout is born.

The Indian health care system is riddled with these touts. They are sometimes the staff working in hospitals, looking to make some extra money. It could be the receptionist, the billing clerk, the ward boy, the liftman, the toilet cleaner, and even the telephone operator. More often, they are professional touts working for doctors and diagnostic facilities but pretending to be a helping hand around sick patients and their worried relatives. One does not have to be a genius mathematician to figure out that each of these touts needs to be successful just a few times in a year for the employers to recover the wages for the whole year.

The more talented and adventurous amongst these develop significant networks within the system and of course do much better. They know how patients turning up at a hospital can be deflected to their patrons. If a certain Dr Singh, in a private hospital in New Delhi, is wondering why nobody ever comes to his clinics, he only needs to send a decoy disguised as a patient to the receptionist in the hospital or to any others who have taken it upon themselves to guide patients in finding somebody whom they can work with. If the hospital reception never puts any patient through to the telephone line in Dr Singh's room, it is possible that the receptionist has been asked to divert all calls to a different number, or it may even be that the telephone ringer is turned off. If you think about it, these people are more ingenious than some of the doctors who occupy these rooms. What a waste of talent though! The management in both private and government institutions knows about these touts who operate in their facilities, but they are helpless. Rather, they pretend to be helpless. The reason is simple. It does not really bother the private hospital which of their consultants gets the patients, as long as they are being seen in the hospital. In fact, if they nurture and support a consultant with an effective (marketing) team, it is more than likely that this person will also pull in business for the hospital from its competitors. Given a choice between ethical doctors who, in the eyes of the management, are lazy sinecures, simply waiting for patients to show up so they can give their professional advice, and doctors who are sufficiently motivated to walk an extra mile to get patients to the hospital and encourage them to get admitted and have operations (sometimes unnecessary), every hospital manager in India knows which one to choose. Health care is a business, and it has to be run like one.

We Indians are not unfamiliar with the world of touts. Visit any government office and you are sure to see a few of them. Processes in Indian bureaucracy are deliberately kept vague, circumstantial and opaque to ensure the survival of touts. Rarely will you find all the information or steps clearly and transparently laid out for you in a brochure or on a website. Even if it is displayed somewhere, it will be in a place where no common man can find it without the help of a tout. Application forms will be out of print, but you can buy them from somebody in the same premises, provided you know where this person can be found. Processes are so designed that your file must pass through a number of hands for a favourable outcome. Each of these noble men and women in the food chain genuinely believes that they are doing their customers a personal favour, for doing a job they are paid to do. Politeness is out of the question and in these fiefdoms of Indian bureaucracy, one can expect to be told off at the slightest hint of misdemeanour. You will be made to run from pillar to post, from one office to another, day after day, until you break down and hire a tout, who will make it all seem so easy that you are left wondering why you didn't do this in the first place.

It probably started with owners of nursing homes and hospitals who cannot survive without a regular stream of patients. Their outgoings are fixed and the business will lose money if each bed does not have a patient in it at any given point of time. (Hospitals use a technical term called bed occupancy rates to express this.) Under these circumstances, it pays to have as large a pool as possible of marketing executives (that is, touts) to tap patients from as wide an area as possible.

Of course, the practice is not just confined to the owners of nursing homes and hospitals anymore. Individual doctors have been quick to arrive on the scene, not wanting to be left out. After all, many doctors know that a commission has to be paid irrespective of who sends the patients. It is actually cheaper to hire these touts and pay off people like the taxi driver or rickshaw-wallah or quacks or RMPs than to strike deals with family doctors who are already being solicited by everyone and usually demand a much higher cut. Most private doctors in India learn soon enough that the solution is not to disengage with the culture of cuts and touts but to inflate your bills to accommodate the additional 'business' expenses. If you ever wondered why private medical health care is so very expensive, now you know it—there are more people involved in the business than you are able to see and there is only one person paying for them all: the patient. The hospital, the doctor, the secretary, the tout, the family doctor, the laboratory owner, the pharmacist, the multinational drug companies—all depend on the patient for survival. As a patient, you are paying not just for your treatment but for all the additional overheads such as the hospital spending crores on hosting a big health care conference, industry sponsorship of your doctor's next holiday trip (oh, should I have said attending a medical conference?) and all of a number of marketing executives, that is, touts, your doctor has hired. If this means hundreds of millions of families cannot even afford basic health care or are pushed into poverty as a result of illness, so be it.

You have to look at these touts as the ships that will help you navigate rough waters. Without their help, you may make it, but only if you are an expert swimmer. Touts know the system. Babus in government offices will not even entertain you because what they can't ask for openly, these touts will do for them. This applies to doctors too. These touts keep our officers and doctors safe from the dirty details. They put themselves in the firing line to protect those sitting in big offices and lavish chambers. A tout is an important cog in the wheel of Indian systems. They help our systems function smoothly despite all the underlying imperfections. The babus who are actually employed to do the job are able to enjoy morning tea in office, read newspapers, and also simultaneously increase their income, while a parallel army of touts does all the work. Doctors are able to concentrate on patients while touts take care of the business of attracting business. Such innovative Indian solutions for Indian problems!

Habdu and his family live in rural Rajasthan, in a little known village some 100 kilometres to the West of Jaipur. Life here is simple. Rain is unpredictable and that means everybody takes up some extra work on the side to survive the times when agriculture is just impossible. Cattle-farming is popular, as are a number of local crafts. Men work hard during the day and spend the evenings outside their mud houses, sitting on cots made of wooden frames and ropes or muddas (chairs made of fine bamboo sticks and ropes), gossiping with each other. Women are usually busy with household chores like washing clothes, milking the cow, preparing cakes of cow dung for fuel and cooking.

Habdu was only in his late fifties but he looked much older. Life hadn't exactly been easy for him and this was obvious to anyone who cared to look at his now frail structure, which had endured the ravages of nature on a daily basis. Each of the wrinkles on his face, the marks on the skin of his feet and legs, and his sparse white hair had a story to tell. Wearing a dhoti that once was white and an even dirtier kurta, he spent his days doing nothing in particular but feeling very busy, productive and important, regardless. After all, he didn't need to do very much. In his part of the world, it was an asset to have sons. With two of them to look after him, Habdu was indeed very lucky and today, he felt it more than the usual.

'Mohan,' he shouted out for one of his sons. 'This cough is not getting better.'

'You should stop smoking, Bauji.'

'It is an old habit, Son. There was no television when we were young and life was tough.'

'Bauji, you will never change. I have heard this story a thousand times. Let us go and see Vaidyaji. His medicines usually work. There is magic in his hands.'

Vaidyaji, as the villagers called him, was the village doctor. He practiced Ayurvedic medicine. He did not have any of the sophisticated knowledge that goes with modern medicine but more than made up for it with his compassion and caring attitude. He rarely asked for anything in return. On occasion, he also dispensed medicines free of cost. If he asked for something, it was never more than a few rupees. People sometimes felt better after taking his medicines; more often, they did not. Nobody ever blamed Vaidyaji though. That was out of question. How could you? Life and death are not in human hands after all. The villagers were always grateful to him and made up with love and gifts what they lacked in money. Everyone in the village respected Vaidyaji and he regularly received gifts in the form of wheat, bajra, vegetables, fruits, sweets, etc. Sometimes, people would go shopping in town, 20 kilometres away from the village. And he would tell them to bring him things that he needed and pay them later. Many a times, the villagers refused to take money.

'Mohan, I don't have a good feeling about it. I think you will have to take him to Jaipur.'

'What do you mean Vaidyaji? Is it serious?'

'Don't tell Habdu anything but I suspect he has got something bad,' Vaidyaji spoke to Mohan in a confidential tone as Habdu was leaving the room.

Vaidyaji had always felt that his job was as much about keeping hope alive as it was about healing patients. He was somewhat economical with the truth but he had found a more satisfactory and less cruel way of dealing with things. He would often share more with the relatives than with the patients themselves.

That evening, a big discussion took place between Habdu's two sons. Money was arranged, responsibilities divided and a plan of action prepared. All Bauji was to be told was that Vaidyaji had advised taking him to Jaipur for a few tests. Besides, he was to be told that money was not an issue. They were worried that if he discovered the family's real financial position, he might just refuse further treatment.

Many rickshaw-wallahs and auto rickshaw drivers at the Sindhi camp bus terminal in Jaipur know more can be made by acting as a commission agent for hospitals and hotels than in their real job. The smart ones amongst them will undercut their peers on the journey fare to make up elsewhere. It is not too difficult to spot a villager who has come to Jaipur for advanced medical treatment. Often, unsuspecting patients will themselves share such details. For what harm could come from sharing your reason for visiting the city with a concerned rickshaw-wallah.

'But why this hospital? This hospital does not have a very good reputation in the city. Since you are from my district, I can take you to a better doctor. If you don't like him, I will take you to your hospital. But you will like this doctor. He is much cheaper and everybody who is treated by him is always cured.'

Such rickshaw-wallahs often arrived at Gupta Nursing home. Dr Gupta had come to Jaipur five years ago and in a relatively short span of time, he had established himself well. The rickshaw-wallah knew Dr Gupta would see him personally and also offer him a cold drink, which he desperately needed after battling the city's sweltering heat.

'What have you got today?' Dr Gupta asked.

'I have a patient,' the rickshaw-wallah said, making himself comfortable in the chair opposite the doctor. He felt no reason to feel inferior to Dr Gupta anymore; he was now a business partner who expected to be treated with respect.

'Have you told him anything?'

'They are expecting some blood tests and a CT scan.'

'Good. Are they well off?'

'They don't look rich but he has a few thousand rupees.'

'OK. Go to the cashier. I heard you took the last patient to Dr Agarwal. Is he giving more these days?'

'What are you saying Doctor Saheb? I only do business with you. I can't help if a patient wants to go to Dr Agarwal.'

'I thought so. After all, we have worked together for so many years now. Anyway, I have increased your commission to 20 per cent from today. Happy?'

Dr Gupta knew that competition was intense and he could not afford to lose any business to his rivals. He had arrived in Jaipur soon after graduation with very little. It had taken a lot of hard work and careful planning to reach where he had. He wasn't going to let go of it now. Many new doctors had settled in the city, he knew. Jaipur was a good city, the only fitting place really for a doctor to raise his family in the whole of Rajasthan. Whereas the rest of the state faced an acute shortage of hospitals and doctors, in Jaipur, the problem was quite the reverse. Most doctors competed for very few patients and hospitals struggled with their profit margins.

In this sense, the problem of health care manpower is not vastly dissimilar to the problem of food shortage in India; it is largely a problem of distribution, not supply. How else can we explain thousands of tonnes of food rotting in ill-equipped government storage facilities? There is no efficient procuring system that can compensate farmers fairly and a distribution system that can take this food to those dying of starvation. This means farmers committing suicides, huge government subsidies on food, colossal grain wastage and hungry poor without the means to buy food all coexist. Similarly, millions of rural and poor Indians cannot afford a doctor, and doctors (and hospitals) in big towns and cities are competing fiercely with each other to attract the very few patients who can afford them.

Without addressing this issue of distribution, creation of more doctors is only exacerbating problems for young doctors in cities without making the lot of people living in remote towns and villages any better. Doctors need good hospitals to work in, good schools to send their children to, facilities for enjoyment and entertainment, and modern housing with electricity, water, telephone and broadband connection. Jaipur offered all of these whereas Habdu's village did not. This is why even those medical students who came from Habdu's district rarely went back to practise there. They were spread out in big cities in different parts of India, and around the world. People from Habdu's district invested in creating such doctors but got nothing in return. New doctors and surgeons arriving in Jaipur had already increased the general practitioners' cut so much that Dr Gupta was struggling to keep up. His marketing team faced a tougher job now. Local family doctors had too many options. He had to think of other ideas to attract business and ensure his survival.

His marketing boys had networked with people working outside bus stands and railways stations. Many pan-wallahs in close vicinity to government and even private hospitals and nursing homes had his visiting card. His team had infiltrated hospitals, both government and private ones. The business model was simple but effective. Commission rates were lower than what the family doctors in the city had begun charging and the pool that his team could tap into was enormous, almost unlimited. He would always have patients, at least until others in the profession figure out his modus operandi. If such a day dawned, he would have to think of newer ways. So he could relax for now, but he could never be complacent.

Others in the city were not going to be left behind. How could they? When survival is at stake, human beings improvise. Isn't it astonishing that people separated by thousands of miles of land and unfathomable vast expanses of water have often travelled a similar journey of innovations and improvisations? So elsewhere in the city, in a big private hospital, Dr Varma was using similar concepts in his hospital practice. He was an orthopaedic surgeon, one of the eight in his hospital. Though hospital machinery worked tirelessly to ensure a regular stream of patients into the hospital, it mattered little to them which of these eight orthopaedic surgeons actually got the patients and did the work. Hospital management knew what was important. Those who had patients, irrespective of how they got them, had an assured place and the support of the hospital.

Dr Varma's secretaries had linked up with the reception staff, lift operators, ward-boys and many other hospital staff to ensure that a large chunk of patients who needed an orthopaedic surgeon came directly to him. Managing such a large number of people within and outside the hospital needed resources. Dr Varma had four secretaries for precisely this purpose. If you understand how difficult this work is, you will surely agree he needed as much help as he could get. Many of his secretaries secretly confided to their friends that he got very upset if he didn't get enough patients. Secretaries could keep their jobs for as long as they could bring patients. How they achieved this was their problem. In doing this, Dr Varma had shifted the responsibility for his own survival down the chain and it had worked.

Unaware of the dealings between doctor and rickshaw-wallah, Habdu and his son waited outside Dr Gupta's air-conditioned chambers in the dry scorching heat of the Jaipur summer. The waiting area was full of people from surrounding villages; poor people in dirty clothes that stuck to their weather-hardened dark, dry skin with white marks left by almost anything that touched it. Most men were dressed in shirts and trousers except the older ones who wore dhoti and kurta. Women wore sarees or ghaghra-cholis with a head scarf that seemed somehow anchored to their head and moved very little as they roamed about. If not the large silver anklets on their feet, the pointed, handmade, embroidered shoes would betray their Rajasthani origin. They had all been brought in by the rickshaw owners from different corners of Jaipur or referred by doctors Dr Gupta had established a good working relationship with in different parts of the state. Some of them occupied the white plastic chairs, almost the same colour now as their white clothes, strewn around the room. Many sat on the floor with their bags; they came prepared in case they had to stay in the city for a few days.

Habdu felt really grateful for having found this helpful rickshaw-wallah, who charged less than the going rate for the trip and also found a really famous doctor (why else would so many people come from all over to see him?). It was nearly lunchtime. Habdu and his son had come prepared with their lunch box.

Dr Gupta's 'chamber' was full of people. One group of patients and relatives were sitting across him in chairs, the other group was around the examination couch with a patient on it, and a third group was trying to attract his attention standing to his right. Dr Gupta and his secretary often had to speak at the top of their voice to manage this crowd. His sharp business sense told him that this created a sense of importance around him which seeing one patient at a time did not. Patients and relatives fought to push themselves to the fore of this crowd to get his attention for even a fleeting moment. This was Dr Gupta's subtle way of telling these people how unimportant they were to his 'business'. Without them, nothing would stop for him. This was the perception he wanted to create, and he had, ever so successfully. Patients felt grateful for each glimpse, each word he spoke, for any bit of advice he gave. He was always very polite, but in the manner people adopt when they know nobody dares to question their authority. He did not need to be rude. Patients and relatives never understood a word of the medical details he patronizingly shared with them, simply to remind them that it was all too technical and they need not worry about it. Patients trusted him implicitly.

Habdu and his son stood sheepishly in the corner of the room, waiting to be called forward. After about ten minutes, they realized they would have to push ahead of the crowd themselves, so they made their way to the premium spot on the right side of Dr Gupta where it was difficult for him to ignore anybody.

'What can I do for you?' offered Dr Gupta politely, pretending not to know anything about them, the conversation with the rickshaw driver fresh in his memory.

'Doctor Saheb, his cough is not showing any sign of stopping for the past two months,' Habdu's son offered.

'Let me see,' Dr Gupta said, rotating his swivel chair towards Habdu and simultaneously gesturing for him to sit on the stool next to him. He always carried a stethoscope around his neck. He put it to his ears and pretended to listen to something. In the noise of the room, it was impossible for him to listen to anything but it was important that he impressed upon the patients the technical nuances of the trade. Over the years, he had discovered that it wasn't even necessary to listen to the chest these days as tests gave you far more information, far more accurately. His patients, however, were not to know this and must continue to believe in his ability to diagnose with his stethoscope.

Dr Gupta scribbled a few illegible lines on his letterhead with an expensive Parker pen, a gift from a pharmaceutical representative. 'Get these tests done. Vinod will take the fees and guide you regarding the rest.' Vinod was his assistant and had been with Dr Gupta for a few years now. The consultation fee was Rs 50 and just to make the deal even sweeter for Habdu, he was told there would be no charge for looking at the reports the next time.

Dr Gupta's wealth was not built on these consultation fees. For at that rate, he would have to see a lot of such patients every day, day after day, to earn a decent living in Jaipur. His family expected him to earn much more. He wanted everyone to know that he was a rich and famous doctor, a very successful doctor. But he could not charge patients more than Rs 50 as consultation fees, for that simply pushed them away. Money still had to be earned. Thankfully, there were ways. Ordering expensive tests from neighbouring diagnostic facilities for a commission and keeping all the five beds in his small nursing home upstairs full all the time were some of these methods.

Tests were not cheap. They needed to be carried out in the centre Dr Gupta's assistant had recommended and they were followed by more tests. Living and commuting in Jaipur, eating in local roadside restaurants, and getting the recommended tests done, all this meant that Habdu's son soon exhausted all that he had brought with him. The money was fully spent and they hadn't even got a diagnosis. Tomorrow, they were told, they would find out what the last rounds of test showed.

'Babaji,' Dr Gupta spoke politely with a hint of compassion and kindness in his voice, 'you know all the bidis you've smoked... That's caused it.'

'Caused what, Doctor Saheb?' asked Habdu's son as his father sat still, waiting for the bad news to follow. Experience had taught him that every act of kindness was usually followed by one of matching cruelty.

'He has got cancer of the lungs. The scan had raised doubts about it but the biopsy confirms it. How much money do you have left?' It was important for Dr Gupta to know this as more money could be made by referring him to a friendly surgeon or oncologist (cancer specialist).

'Tests are so expensive, Doctor Saheb. We have spent most of what we had brought with us,' Habdu said, before his son could open his mouth. Habdu knew instinctively that he had to save his family from any further expenditure on his health. The cancer was his fault and others in the family should not be made to suffer for it.

'I suspected that,' Dr Gupta said in a caring tone, 'take this referral letter to City Government Hospital. It is much cheaper there.'

Difficulties faced by the patients in City Government Hospital are of a different nature. Doctors there don't have to resort to any of the tactics their private counterparts use to lure patients. With corridors and wards full of patients and relatives also doubling up as attendants, there is no shortage of patients here. In fact, every single hospital facility is overstretched to an extreme, trying to meet the exponentially increasing demand. Since the hospital is completely government owned and funded, it provides the power-hungry officials in the state health department a strong lever to micro-manage the day-to-day affairs of the hospital, ensuring the hospital administration occupy merely symbolic positions. They cannot take any major decision, build for the future, appoint to any significant position without interference from the political and bureaucratic masters, remove any member of staff for fear of retaliation from the unions, raise their own finances, or even use their alumni network to promote their institution. The entire administration is riddled with red tape, nepotism, inefficiency and blatant corruption. Most of the government fund that this hospital gets is spent on paying the wages of thousands of people. There is little left to rebuild the decaying infrastructure, buy the latest equipment for doctors or build modern comfortable facilities for patients. Poor patients (and it is only those who cannot afford to go to private facilities who come here) find themselves coping with the challenges of sickness, poverty, illiteracy and bureaucracy, all at the same time. They are desperate for help and they will take it from anybody.

Government hospitals and poor unsuspecting patients filling these premises are ideal hunting grounds for predatory touts. They appear as saviours, who can help you navigate these ancient buildings and their equally archaic administrative procedures. They can take you to the right doctor, bypass a queue, get a test done quicker, find a hospital bed when doctors have told you there is none, and even find a place for your family to be put up in if you are new to Jaipur—all for a small sum of money. Taking a purely market perspective, these individuals fill an important gap in the market. Without these touts, many patients would simply have nowhere to go. However, these touts are not really altruistic angels. Many of them are agents for hospital staff and doctors, much like the touts working for babus in the vast Indian bureaucracy. Some work for local diagnostic centres and private hospitals. Some others are actually hospital staff who can use their connections with doctors (who also get a share of the commission) to help you bypass a queue for diagnostic tests or a hospital bed.

Habdu will soon lose the money 'spared' by Dr Gupta to one of these touts. More tests will be carried out in yet another private facility and finally, doctors will declare his cancer incurable. Habdu will return to die in his village, his family poorer but none the wiser. Of course, they remain grateful to the rickshaw driver, Dr Gupta and the tout for all the help they received in Jaipur. That this help did not change the outcome does not bother people who have learnt to leave everything to God. The insurmountable difficulties of life usually enhance people's faith in the supreme power. God wins each time humanity fails.

Patients: Be Aware

Though savvier patients and relatives already know of the commission culture and will not go to the laboratory or hospital recommended by the family doctor, what they don't know is that it makes no difference. The laboratory or hospital will not pass on the savings to them unless they insist on a discount. In many cases, the mere fact that your doctor has phoned the hospital to say that you are his client will be sufficient to set off a commission trail. Just like when I visited Darjeeling many years ago, the hotel owner told me that the very fact that I arrived in a taxi means that the commission is now due to the taxi owner if I stayed in his hotel.

Even the most aware patients will find it difficult to identify touts in all the various avatars they can take. In the Indian health care industry, there are very few people who will be moved by the sight of a sick or poor patient, and anybody pretending to help you is doing just that. Patients need to be aware of this simple fact. These days, information about most doctors is easily available on the Internet and my recommendation would be to explore your options before you visit the hospital or nursing home. It is best to speak to doctors directly and, if possible, see them in a private clinic free of these external influences. If you are going to visit a hospital, it is important not to listen to anybody whilst in the premises, as any person could be an agent of some other doctor or hospital. Short of a major media campaign, I cannot think of any other way to take this message out to the masses.

Government Facilities: Take a Consumer-Centric Approach

Navigating the corridors of our public health care system is impossible for even a fit, educated person. An ill, uneducated, poor person then simply has no chance. It is not beyond human will to come up with practical suggestions to improve information sharing in public health care. It can't be impossible to share with patients transparently the state of beds in the hospital, or the patient's number on the waiting list for tests and treatments. It is surely not beyond human ability to have proper signposts for all of the hundreds of doctors and departments. Why can't we have leaflets printed in patients' language, and reception staff who are polite? Government machinery in India needs a cultural change and that can only happen when there are effective complaint mechanisms for patients to report the corrupt, the rude and the incompetent. Our public hospital machinery often forgets that they are here to serve patients and helping patients is their job, not a favour. Even seventy years after Independence, the colonial mind-set of the bureaucracy is showing little signs of change. They still work for their masters and not the people.

Hospitals: Manage Your Premises

If you ask any hospital manager about the existence of touts on their premises, first, they will deny it and then gradually, they will pretend helplessness. For private hospitals, touts are only a problem if they take business away from the hospitals. If a tout in a private hospital directs a patient from one doctor to the other, the hospital loses nothing. In government hospitals, many officials and doctors are often hand in glove with these touts.

I find it interesting when hospitals say they have no control over who gets into their premises. If they don't, who does? Should they not have a stricter system in place to ensure that only genuine patients and their relatives get in and nobody else? Is it not the responsibility of the hospitals to secure their premises? It will only take a few surprise checks followed by handing over of a few touts to the police and prosecution of a few laboratory and nursing home owners to bring about an abrupt halt to this practice in government hospitals. For private hospitals with their armies of security personnel, the job should be even easier.

Regulatory authorities could also help with some surprise checks. Doctors found to be hiring them should be permanently erased from the medical register and the licences of laboratories and hospitals using touts permanently suspended.

Patients Cannot Have It Both Ways

We have a choice. When your mother needs blood, are you going to donate it yourself or buy it from somewhere? When your brother is dying of kidney failure, would you rather find a donor from within the family or pay five lakh rupees to buy one? I have heard many businessmen and government officers complain bitterly about the declining values in the medical profession in India but the same people don't think tax evasion or bribery in their own work sphere are serious issues worth talking about. We all want to see others improve first.

If you want good, honest doctors, you have to pay them a fair fee and due respect. You have to ensure you keep your appointment and if unable to do so, offer an apology and pay for wasted time. Doctors are not shopkeepers. If you are going to shop around, you will turn them into one. Today in India, the foundations of the noble doctor–patient relationship are shaken and though the majority of the blame lies with the doctors, patients too could do with some introspection.

Population Explosion

Let us not forget the root cause of a number of these problems. The reason we have a large number of touts willing to engage in frankly illegal, immoral behaviour is because we have a significantly large section of very poor population desperate to earn a livelihood. When it comes to the survival of his family, what will a man not do? The reason we cannot have an adequate public health care system in place to look after the needs of the entire population of the country is because no government in the world, not even the richest, can take complete ownership for such massive numbers. India is developing, but our population and its needs are growing more rapidly. I agree that education is a good contraceptive, but a mandatory one-child policy enforced by a willing and well-meaning state could be a better contraceptive and one likely to yield quicker results.

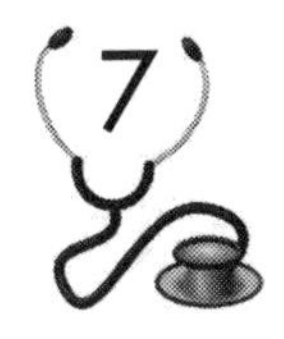

False Claims

Nearly 72 per cent of IVF clinics made exaggerated claims by promising certain pregnancy.

—The *Times of India*, Ahmedabad, 6 June 2015

Current consent procedures seem inadequate as a means for the expression of autonomous choice and their ethical standing can be called into question.

—Rajesh DR et al in *Journal of Indian Academy of Forensic Medicine*, Volume 35(1):40-3

It is a difficult balance to achieve. You leave things to the markets and they are prone to greed and excesses. You nationalize them and this usually means inefficiency and corruption. Societies continually swing back and forth between these two choices, and India is no exception. Government systems need transparency, accountability and commitment to public service; private ones need monitoring and control by strong regulatory bodies. When it comes to health care, all of these are sadly missing. Government systems suffer from lack of vision and planning in addition to financial constraints, bureaucratic red tape, vested interests and corruption. Private systems stand accused of unethical practices, business-like culture and absence of the ethos of service. Individual doctors with nowhere to go are caught in the middle. Government facilities are so poorly equipped and inadequate for the purpose that job satisfaction is little. Private hospitals have to focus on money to be sustainable and generate profits for shareholders. You go freelance and you are competing with your fellow colleagues and professionals for work.

Given these dynamics, individual doctors feel the obvious need to ensure that patients not only come to them for treatment but also believe that they are the best doctors in the field. How do they go about achieving this? They could, of course, just hope that if they keep doing good work, sooner or later, word will go around and they will have some patients. However, they have bills to pay today, and that people will actually ever find out their real worth cannot be guaranteed. At the same time, there are many well-recognized tricks that work effectively and can create an aura of success and fame around them. The choice is rather simple. They could opt for a lifetime of struggle and earn the tag of being complacent and laidback from friends and family; or they could be a bit proactive about it, and the fame, money and glory could be theirs for the taking.

Third Party Endorsement

We talked about advertising in Chapter 1 and we saw how businesses are allowed to advertise whereas doctors are not. This means doctors are better off either launching a business or working for one, to improve their visibility. For the rest, there are other time-tested tricks. One that works most effectively is to get somebody else to say you are the best. The value of independent, unbiased third party confirmation and endorsement is entrenched in human civilization. When it comes to health care, such endorsement can be bought, depending on your willingness to engage with the system of cut practice and commissions. Increase your commission rates and you convince your general practitioners why you are the person they should send patients to. And how will they convince a patient to go to you only? Your virtues will be extolled and your reputation boosted. Overnight, you will become 'the best in the city' and 'world famous'. The alternative is hard work for an indefinite period of time with no guarantee of success.

The Globetrotter

Almost every doctor knows that if you are constantly travelling all over the world (on account of drug and equipment companies or corporate hospitals of course), it will be much easier to earn the tag of success. Such tactics work elegantly for patients who hold 'globetrotting' doctors in high esteem. I remember a patient boasting, 'You can never get hold of my surgeon. He is always abroad.' One would think patients would prefer doctors who have time for them!

A renowned surgeon in Delhi was recently quoted as saying this, 'Mr Agarwal, please look around and see all these people. Do you really think I am bothered if you don't get this operation done by me? How much do you think I earn in a day?' This was followed by claims of personal wealth and earning that would put business tycoons to shame. Mr Agarwal, very rich himself, must have felt his personal wealth and existence to be of no consequence in front of such a doctor. It is common knowledge amongst private practitioners in India that a polite, caring attitude is often misinterpreted by Indian patients as a doctor 'too keen' and it actually drives them away. A little bit of disrespect and off-handedness measured carefully and delivered astutely can go a long way in such an environment.

One proud patient spoke to me about his very famous and successful surgeon in these terms: 'There are always a large number of people waiting to see him, like the crowds outside Mata's temple, and he sometimes sees a few patients at the same time.' Now please help me understand this. What is the link between poor management of patient flow and success? Of course, doctors understand the psychology of patients well. Why would you hire a secretary to manage your appointment timings, risk a patient not turning up at all, provide privacy, give patients your undivided attention, and yet, in the end, create an impression that you are not popular or successful?

Fake Degrees

Recognized academic qualifications matter. They indicate competence and generate patient confidence. Each of the letters that follow your doctor's name on his certificates indicates talent and years of toil and sweat. However, when nobody is watching and nobody can tell the difference, nothing can prevent anybody from adding a few titles to their name. It is not at all uncommon for quacks to don fake titles or invent new ones that mean nothing. Lately, even qualified doctors are seen displaying certificates and memberships that don't mean much. They could attend a course for a few days and obtain a few additional letters to add after their name. If the qualification mentions the name of a Western institution, it will impress patients even more. Western institutions also know it and they are only too happy to let you use their credentials and name as long as you can pay a fee, sometimes an annual fee for continued use of the privilege. It is a different matter altogether that many doctors then stop paying subscriptions and continue to use the title long after the accrediting body has erased their name for non-payment of annual membership fees. Many doctors invent new qualifications and many prominently display visits and short-term fellowships at famous centres as certification of their expertise.

Yes, authorities could clamp down on these doctors but what can they do when a large number of doctors are indulging in unethical or illegal behaviour? Should we make a criminal of all of them or should we tone down the regulations? These are profound questions that go right to the heart of modern Indian society, and not just the health care system.

Invited Lectures and Medical Conferences

Really famous doctors must also deliver invited lectures to august audiences. There is nothing wrong with it too. If you have worked hard all your life, written a few good papers and found a thing or two, it is only logical that you share your findings with others. A majority of private doctors in India have little time or interest, beyond what is required to ensure a constant flow of patients (and money), to engage in serious academic stuff. In such an environment, invitations to lectures at meetings don't depend on your academic proficiency but on your ability to return the favour.

Essentially, if you expect to be invited to conferences, you have to do the same in turn. This obviously does not include the real and genuine academics out there as very few private doctors in India belong to this category. Doctors know that it will be easier to climb up the ranks if they are constantly lecturing around the globe and occupy prestigious positions on the boards of various societies. Any impression that you are a world-class academic, even if it is false, will go a long way in boosting your local reputation and business.

Organizing a medical conference is no joke either. In most countries, this is the job of big societies, the ones that represent the professionals of the country. As we have seen elsewhere in this book when discussing continuing medical education, these conferences should only be allowed to go on as long as the expenses are kept under control and the ethos of sharing and learning do not degenerate into five-star parties. In India, if you are a big doctor worth your name, you must hold conferences periodically, and invite friends and colleagues from the rest of the country and abroad. They will do the same for you and this will ultimately become a closed club of conference organizers offering enhanced professional visibility, success and fame. Especially in these days of Facebook and Twitter, when every single action can easily be broadcast to potential patients (read business), these activities are very important. Even public sector doctors, who do not always stand to benefit from increased patient flow, are attracted by the enhanced professional and social reputation on offer, something that may translate into a financially more successful private practice tomorrow. With so many of these events being organized regularly nowadays, the organizers need to go out of their way to attract attendees and audiences. They must ensure all the needs of the delegates are met. Obviously, a comfortable setting and a good meal will be useful. Live operating can further add to the excitement. Star speakers from around the globe on paid trips pulls in more crowds, and if you can manage a real celebrity, this could even lure the local media into covering the conference.

The practice of organizing medical conferences must be good for business, as I often hear famous private doctors boasting about how much they have spent from their own pocket towards such events. In one particular conversation I recall, a surgeon spent fifteen lakh rupees from his own pocket to hold a major annual conference on behalf of a society of surgeons. I think this is an issue for the regulators to address. The need for continued professional education must be balanced against the expenses involved, for after all it is the patients who ultimately end up footing these expenses.

The Inventor in the News

On top of all this, if a doctor is also a pioneer—an inventor, an innovator—then he could even persuade the local press to sing his praises, and that can be really good for business. The medical regulator in India is weak; patients are largely unaware. There is no monitoring of individual doctor performance. Competition for the top slot is fierce and the media is always looking for breakthroughs. In such an environment, doctors know that doing anything different or new can propel them into limelight straightaway. It does not matter if the invention is actually good or has gone through scientific scrutiny. It also does not matter if appropriate ethical safeguards had been taken and patients informed of the potential risks. As long as it is something new, irrespective of need and merit, the media is all too happy to broadcast it.

Science journalists in developed countries usually have a deep understanding of the subject matter themselves and rarely report things not published in reputed medical journals. Now, I am a passionate advocate for freedom of expression of scientists in scientific fora, and it is my belief that scientists from developing countries are disadvantaged by current publishing paradigms and systems. However, to put every new development in the public domain before the scientific community has had a chance to examine it will not correct this problem. The media is well advised to stay away from new medical advances until they have been validated. Next time you read something about a 'world's first' in a newspaper, perhaps you should question if it has gone through some scientific scrutiny and if not, why? World over, scientists only discuss results with the media after publication in scientific journals. If an Indian doctor shares details of an innovative operation with the *Times of India* instead of the *National Medical Journal of India*, it is only logical that questions are asked.

It is also true that without the help of an expert in public relations, you will not be able to get local media to cover your activities and broadcast them. We live in a world where news is often made, but only sometimes reported. You may be the best surgeon in the world but if you can't get local newspapers to interview you, carry your quotes, or talk about you, you'll never become truly famous. Journalists are looking for stories and if you have operated on a celebrity, it is in your interest to ensure that the news gets out (leaked). This is the fastest route to fame. Recently, a friend of mine was asked by a journalist if he had operated on any famous patient. It did not matter to this journalist that in divulging those details, my friend might be violating the confidence embodied in a doctor–patient relationship. But can we really blame the media when many doctors themselves leak the news of treating a celebrity? Can we really blame doctors when leaking such news is the best way of becoming a celebrity themselves?

Too Much Information

I remember a surgeon telling me that the medical director of his hospital asked him not to 'overwhelm' patients with 'information overload'. After all, Indian patients should expect to be patronized. You must promise complete cure without any ifs and buts. Just decide what is best for them (usually it means deciding what is best for you or your hospital) and do it. You only need to walk through any town or city in India to know where to get 'guaranteed' cure for your piles, lack of libido, sexual problems, infertility, etc. And if you are looking for the most experienced surgeon in the world, you need look no further. They have all performed thousands of procedures with a 100 per cent success rate. It does not really matter if there is no verifiable record of such information or if the doctors themselves have no idea about how many procedures they have performed with what success rate. Patients only want to go to the most experienced surgeon in the world and each surgeon knows that that search must end with them. Practising medicine in India is an art where grooming patients needs to be learnt along with the ability to operate upon them. You could survive without the latter, but not the former.

The Search for the Best

Imagine there are fifty doctors in a small town. How do they reach out to the public and other doctors in the area? For a patient, what are the available mechanisms to find a doctor with specialized interest in a specific medical condition and to know about his/her results in that field? The doctor–patient relationship in India has now fallen so low that patients have, for want of options, become consummate consumers. It is rare for patients to go with the advice of a single clinician when it comes to major or expensive medical decisions. If the advice of the second doctor is in conflict with that of the first one, they will go and see a third one. The final decision is arbitrary, based on a number of emotional and generally illogical parameters.

Fear is a strong emotion and some doctors know how to use it to retain patients. For example, a doctor says that you face imminent and untimely death from a heart attack if you don't get a coronary stent today. Would you at this point really listen to other doctors who may assure you that everything is all right? What if the first doctor is correct? There is another aspect worth examining. The patient involved may be your father who is depending on you not just to pay the medical bills but also to make the right choice. If you walked away from the stenting, what will your father think? Many doctors know well the emotional dynamics and family psychology that rule the Indian psyche and will not hesitate to use this knowledge to enhance their income.

An Indian-born British surgeon I know personally recently visited India to be with his dying 85-year-old mother. 'She was dying. They knew it well. But they still kept her in the ICU for three weeks to extract money from us. All my brothers and sisters were there but knowing their financial condition, I knew I would be the one paying the bills and of course, I was happy to do it for my mother. But you know, she really suffered. If she was my patient, I would just have kept her comfortable and let things take their course. But she was not. She was my mother. The doctors trusted to make things easier for her in her last few days let her down. They knew that the family would never ask them to discontinue treatment. If I said something, it would appear that I just wanted to save some money. So I kept quiet.'

Medical advice needs to be both scientific and compassionate. Yes, sometimes a treatment worth lakhs of rupees can prolong the life of a terminally ill cancer patient by three months but if this means that the family will end up selling their house, the compassionate advice to the family may well be to forgo the treatment and concentrate on easing the pain and suffering of the diseased. However, it is not uncommon for oncologists in India to keep treating cancer patients with one expensive drug after another until the patient is dead and the whole family has been brought to their knees, financially and emotionally. This is why I strongly feel that societies must find a way to separate day-to-day medical decisions from financial incentives. When we incentivize doctors to make people ill, it is a matter of time before the whole population will be declared ill one way or the other. We see this happening already. Aren't we all now suffering from one disease or the other? The human body is a machine and as it grows old, it may develop flaws. In my opinion, only the bigger flaws need addressing and minor wear and tear can usually be safely ignored. The problem is none of us are now allowed to live with even the slightest of variations outside normal parameters. Health care is an industry and this industry benefits if all of us are ill.

It is not too hard to define a good doctor: somebody who understands medical science, has the time to talk to patients, understands patients' issues, and treats them with scientific, evidence-based medicine, delivered in a comfortable environment, with a kind, compassionate attitude. As a medical student, I used to think famous doctors are good doctors who embody these traits. In fact, I remember agreeing with a friend of mine who once remarked about a specialist in Kolkata, 'If he is so good, why isn't he famous?' Twenty-four years later, my opinion is different. Now I know famous doctors are not always the best doctors. And to be completely honest, I will say the best doctors in today's India are probably not famous at all. Those who are famous simply know how to create that impression successfully.

From a patient's perspective, what are the mechanisms to separate the best from the rest? This is a fundamental question, but one that I believe would not need answering if we were able to guarantee competence with qualifications. Currently, patients know that every doctor may have the qualification but not every doctor has the necessary education and training that goes with it.

I can understand why patients constantly look for (but rarely find) an honest, competent doctor. They go from doctor to doctor in this search. But little do patients know that nowhere in the world can you accurately compare two doctors. In the West, there is some movement towards making performance data of doctors public but, even there, it will be some time before we get an accurate assessment of doctors' competence based on their previous performance. A good doctor has a number of attributes. Academic knowledge, application skill, ability to work hard and at odd hours, ability to think on his feet, staying up-to-date dexterity, technical skills, compassion, kindness, sound communication, good judgment ... these are some of the qualities that a doctor needs to have. It will indeed take a very complex algorithm to take them all into account and come up with a numerical rating for a doctor. It is my opinion that in a country like ours, it is simply impossible to tell competent doctors from the not-so-competent ones. The public must understand this and not let marketing decibels or paid mouthpieces of 'famous' doctors undermine the efforts of hard-working, dedicated doctors who are simply doing a good job without knowing how to market themselves to get public attention. If we continue to seek the loudest and the most famous, then as patients, we are doing a disservice to the medical profession, the society, and eventually, to ourselves.

Public Recognition and Awards

A doctor from a big city recently wrote to me saying that he was offered an award by a UK agency but there was a fee for it, so could I check that the agency was genuine? The doctor wasn't sure what the award was for. However, this did not prevent him from paying the money to claim it. 'It would look good in the clinic,' he said. Besides, this was an authentic award being given by an authentic Western agency. Nobody would ever know about the payment.

In a world where, periodically, the political establishment even in developed countries stands accused of selling honours for cash, how difficult is it for doctors and hospitals to influence the handing out of awards and medals? Starting from small local medical association awards to even national awards at times, they can all be influenced depending on whom one knows and what one is willing to pay in return. I am not suggesting all awards are fake and undeserved, just that we should learn to not take everything that attracts us at face value. The best doctors, who are busy day and night, helping and treating patients, don't always have the time to roam around the world on an industry budget or network to obtain awards.

It is not my intention to undermine the entire system of recognition in the country as I am sure a large number of awards do go to the right person, but I simply want us to bear in mind that the parameters of our search for best doctors need to be broadened so as to not exclude the most deserving. At the same time, we must be armed with a healthy dose of scepticism so that we may look beneath the surface, see beyond the obvious. My aim is to expose those who simply know how to market themselves without any real talent and to strengthen the hard-working, dedicated lot who need our support to make an honest living. I want to ensure that the next time anyone is looking for a good doctor, they know where to look and how to look.

Don't Shop for the Best

Doctors undergo a long and arduous journey right from the beginning of their career. Sound academic background, years of training, scores of examinations and long periods of apprenticeships in low paid jobs contribute to the making of a typical Indian doctor. Is it then fair to also expect them to have to market themselves to earn a living? This unnecessary pressure to establish a market presence forces doctors to lie to patients and make claims that are either unscientific or unethical or untrue. And it hinders them from cultivating the true qualities of a good doctor—good clinical outcomes, research, teaching and training.

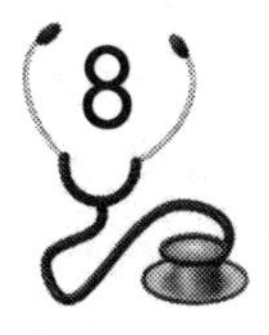

The Quacks

In rural Madhya Pradesh, only 11 per cent of health care providers who were sampled reported having a medical degree, and just over half reported some education beyond high school.

—Jishnu Das et al, Senior Economist,
World Bank, Health Affairs

It is estimated that about 10 lakh quacks are practicing Allopathic medicine, out of which 4 lakh belong to practitioners of Indian Medicine.

—Indian Medical Association

It is not an easy problem to solve. With 0.7 doctors per 1, 000 population compared to 2.5 in the UK and 2.8 in the US, India simply does not have enough doctors to look after its 1.2 billion plus people. The problem is further compounded with most of the nearly 7,00,000 doctors in India being concentrated in urban India, for very good reason of course.

Of these, approximately 1,00,000 doctors work in the public sector and only a third of government doctors work in the rural areas, where two-thirds of our population lives. Overall, rural India has approximately 1 doctor for every 25,000 people. The problem is particularly acute when it comes to primary care. Government primary health centres do not have adequate infrastructure and the underpaid doctors here are either absent from work or so overburdened and disillusioned by the system that they have become ineffective. Private doctors, on the other hand, want the kind of remuneration that most rural patients are unable to pay. Job satisfaction amongst both private and public sector doctors in India is so low that it is hardly surprising they want money to compensate for it. Western countries provide doctors opportunities to excel in many areas such as research, academics, training, management, leadership, and so on; as a result, money is not their only goal. In India, money is the only benchmark for professionals—the only method for them to convince the rest of the world that they are good, that they are better than the ordinary. This hinders any real provision of health care for the majority of the population thanks to a misdirected and demoralized force. Excellence achieved in this environment is then an individual trait, not a systematic phenomenon.

Given this scenario, do you really blame the poor when they turn to quacks for their health care needs? If a patient cannot afford even a quack, he will take advice from the shop assistant in pharmacy shops, or he will self-medicate. I am not denying that cultural mores play a role too. In a blindly religious society, it is common to see an illness treated as an act of God, its outcome best left in His hands.

The Qualified Quack

Before we turn on the real quacks, we must spend some time understanding the qualified quacks. A medical qualification is a desirable commodity within a global market. Competition for the limited seats in government-owned medical colleges can be intense and this has led to mushrooming of private medical colleges. These institutions cater to those willing to pay a price for a medical degree. They do not take public money and help create the much-needed human resources. The arrangement can be mutually beneficial and the doctors created in these institutions can add value to society as long as the entry and exit barriers are appropriately set. Many of us have rehearsed these arguments *ad nauseam* during 'caste reservation' debates. Just as we cannot use the argument that there is 'somebody better out there' against reservation for sections socially ostracized for millennia, we cannot take away the right to self-educate from those who have the means. Moreover, opening a large number of private institutions without addressing the shortage of teaching faculty and postgraduate training places for doctors created in these institutions simply creates more problems than it solves.

It will not really serve anybody's needs, certainly not that of the patients, if these institutions were to accept those who could not stand the rigours of medical training and lack the talent needed to absorb it. Society will be none the richer and the doctors produced will have the qualification but not the ability. These issues would be irrelevant if we could ensure that students entering all medical colleges, government or private, reserved category or not, male or female, satisfy a commonly accepted set of admission criteria, undergo well structured education and training, and are judged to have met adequate course completion standards via a robust exit examination.

These 'minor' safeguards are sometimes ignored in contemporary India in our zeal to look after the marginalized sections of society. We become so fair to the economically disadvantaged and the minorities that we are not fair to the ordinary mainstream citizens. Broadly, this should mean limiting numbers of the marginal categories so that they do not impinge on the rights of the mainstream where merit must rule the roost. For example, reserving more than say 15 per cent of seats in government medical colleges for disadvantaged sections of society might just ensure that a different section of community is being prepared for the disadvantaged tag in future. Marginalizing the mainstream will not bring the marginalized to the mainstream. This simple fact of life seems beyond the grasp of our leaders who remain entrenched in vote bank politics.

There are approximately 12,000 positions for postgraduate training for some 30,000 doctors who qualify each year. The rest are left to fend for themselves without any opportunity for further training or a job. Even for those who do successfully get into a postgraduate training programme, there are no mechanisms to ascertain that training being imparted does indeed meet satisfactory standards. As a result, thousands of these doctors leave for countries like USA, UK, Australia and Canada where they find opportunities for further structured training over many years in reasonably paid jobs. You can do the calculations. How are these countries able to provide jobs to these young doctors while we cannot? They obviously have more jobs for junior doctors than the number of graduates they produce themselves. Given the fact that junior doctors play a vital role in running any hospital, it is not impossible for us to work out a mechanism where private hospitals could be involved in training junior doctors systematically. We could have a national system, similar to the Resident Matching programmes in the US, where each hospital offers a number of training places and doctors keen on further postgraduate training could be 'matched' with the most suitable 'programme'. This would be a win-win situation. Currently, private hospitals and clinics struggle to attract juniors and a large number of doctors have no opportunity for further post-graduate training.

Though postgraduate medical education and training in India is generally in need of significant reformation and reinforcement, nowhere else is this need felt more strongly than in primary care. There is currently no structured training programme for those wishing to become general practitioners, even though this is what most doctors will end up doing. This is despite the widespread recognition that it requires further training over many years before a freshly graduated doctor can comfortably treat patients independently, without any supervision. Acquiring knowledge from textbooks is one thing; applying it in the real world is another. The current scenario in India, where these young professionals are left to engender their own training as well as earn a livelihood, lies at the root of many ethical and practical challenges the medical profession faces today. Doctors spend many years working in private and government hospitals and medical centres, hoping to acquire knowledge that they will one day be able to use in their eventual career as a general practitioner. The training they receive in hospitals is often not fit for this purpose, as they will practice in a different environment in the community, one that will certainly not be structured with any definite exit point. It is very much a case of when you feel ready to take the plunge to practise on your own. If you feel that doctors today behave like businessmen, it is worth sparing a thought for the options that we as a society are leaving them with. When these young professionals do take the plunge in the real world out there, with no secure income and a family with expectations, will they not use all the means at their disposal to find a niche for themselves in the marketplace? The bitterness of this struggle never leaves them as they grow into mature professionals with little sense of gratitude towards the wider society.

Even for those who are lucky enough to competitively secure the few places for postgraduate specialist training that there are in the country, there is no guarantee that they will leave the medical colleges and institutions with the required skills and knowledge. When it comes to medical qualifications, postgraduate training is where the gap between India and the rest of the world really widens. The gap is widest in surgical and interventional specialties where training is most difficult and the lack of it most obvious. What you get at the end of the training is not a specialist who can function independently, rather a doctor who has obtained the degrees to follow his name but not necessarily the skills to match them.

This problem is further aggravated by doctors practising outside their field of expertise. In a business-driven culture, no doctor wants to let go of a patient, irrespective of his ability to treat the patient's condition. It is not uncommon to hear stories of general practitioners performing appendicectomies (operation to remove the appendix) or other operations they are not trained to perform. Then we also hear of 'ghost' surgeons, who perform the actual operation but the family or the patient never sees them. It will take a further chapter to explain why a qualified surgeon might wish to work as a ghost surgeon for a fraction of the fee and let somebody else take the credit for his work. On the face of it, the arrangement is somewhat similar to a particular branded 'showroom' selling goods manufactured under other brands. The underlying drivers are also similar. After all, it is much better for a young surgeon to stay in practice and earn something than lose both money and, eventually, skill.

Even in big corporate hospitals, it is not uncommon to see a patient being admitted under a doctor of a completely different specialty from the one that he needs, depending on a number of factors and 'arrangements'. Doctors affiliated to private hospitals usually learn very quickly how important it is to maintain a good relationship with admitting doctors and administrative staff, if they want a steady flow of patients under them. Unsuspecting patients are being duped every step of their journey.

The exact extent of prevalence of such practices is impossible to estimate but most doctors know these things happen and have given in. No one individual can even attempt to change the direction of this stream without drowning in it. Politicians, whose job it is to do something about this situation, have other, more pressing priorities, such as how to fund their next election campaign. To be able to find a doctor fit for the purpose, properly qualified and adequately trained, is a matter of chance and luck in India. And these are the real doctors in society, the ones who have obtained the necessary qualifications.

The Quacks

A quack refers to a person who does not have any knowledge of any particular system of medicine but still practices in that system. One of the biggest problems in our medical establishment is that there is little control over who can treat patients using the modern (Allopathic) system of medicine. It is even said that India has more quacks than doctors, the approximate numbers being 1 and 0.7 million respectively.

The AYUSH Practitioners

AYUSH is an acronym to denote practitioners of Ayurveda, Yoga and Naturopathy, Unani System, Siddha System and Homeopathy.

Now I believe Allopathic/ modern medicine to be the only established form of scientific medicine recognized and practised around the world. In this context, my competing interests as a practitioner of Allopathic/modern medicine and a general/ bariatric surgeon must be disclosed. Allopathic medicine has now evolved as the only inclusive, evidence-based system of medicine. It includes any treatment within its fold as long as it has been proved to be effective, irrespective of the system and culture it originates from. There are many examples of medicines and surgical practices once used by practitioners of traditional systems that are now incorporated in mainstream medical science.

My views on these systems of medicine notwithstanding, I have no problem with patients seeing a practitioner of Ayurvedic medicine if that is who they want to see, but consulting an Ayurveda practitioner while believing that one is consulting an MBBS doctor qualified in modern medicine is a matter of honesty. One cannot fault those practitioners of traditional systems who clearly mention in writing outside their clinics regarding the system they practice in, who audit their results and do not indulge in prescribing modern medicine. The problem lies with those who write 'Doctor' outside their clinic, don't declare their area of expertise transparently, and end up dispensing potions containing common Allopathic drugs, or sometimes even blatantly prescribe them. Though in a country where even doctors qualified in modern medicines, sometimes prescribe Ayurvedic medicines and are able to invent more letters to write after their names than universities can give out, to expect complete honesty from practitioners of traditional medicine is a tough ask.

One does not wish to dismiss traditional systems of medicine. These systems have evolved over centuries and contain innumerable hidden pearls of wisdom. Ignoring them completely will be overlooking and disregarding our own ancestral heritage. At the same time, blindly following traditional remedies is not likely to convince the world that we are not merely a mystical land of elephant keepers and snake charmers anymore. What is needed is proper research into our traditional remedies. If the Indian government is really serious about finding a place for our traditional systems of medicine in global medical literature, it needs to start investing heavily in research. Identifying active ingredients from some of these traditional remedies, testing them out in trials and then rolling them out for use is possible, but it is going to be neither cheap nor easy.

Religious Healers or 'Babas'

India is a deeply religious country and it is not uncommon for the ill and the suffering to turn to religion when all else has failed. There are a variety of religious and faith-based healers—the babas—engaged in the business of miracle cure. They are even more difficult to deal with than quacks. As we see from time to time, it is not too difficult to stir up religious passions in the country and if you are going to engage in any illegal activity, you are best advised to give it some sort of a religious dimension. This will then paralyse our political and judicial establishment completely. Our babas can preach any treatment to millions in the guise of religious doctrines, and nobody will dare question them. It may harm millions of patients but the whole of society will watch like mute and powerless spectators. The MCI cannot do anything to them as they are not doctors and do not come under their purview. (That it does not do much to monitor qualified doctors either is a different matter altogether.) The police is powerless as most of these religious healers have very strong connections in the political establishment of the country. Politicians, religious leaders, criminals ... in India, sometimes it is difficult to tell the difference.

Registered Medical Practitioners (RMPs)

From time to time, many states in India have advocated and created a separate cadre of paramedical work force, loosely brought under an umbrella term of RMP (Registered Medical Practitioner). There is obvious confusion in the name, because if these people are registered medical practitioners, what are doctors? Sometimes, RMP is used to indicate Rural Medical Practitioner. The term PMP (Private Medical Practitioner) also exists. These are people from various backgrounds who have been given limited licence to practise medicine. Many of these certificates have been issued by state governments, others by a number of institutions of dubious credibility. Usually, these are people who have obtained some medical training in a clinic, health centre or hospital. Some of these are trained in AYUSH specialties. Though there is significant variation in what they are allowed to do, the idea is to deploy them to promote preventive health care and first aid in areas not served by doctors, that is, in rural areas and urban slums. They are not allowed to prescribe 'scheduled' drugs, or dispense anything other than Over-The-Counter (OTC) medicines, and are certainly not allowed to call themselves 'doctors'. However, these are precisely the sorts of things most of them will ultimately indulge in. Many RMPs work as full-fledged doctors and benefit greatly from the cut practice culture.

Quacks Are Not Cheap

Though there are quacks out there pretending to be doctors with elaborate systems, clinics, even hospitals in place, I think a majority of them do not pretend, really speaking. People know whom they are going to but have no choice, as they simply cannot afford the real doctors. What people do not know is that our quacks are not cheap either. Most of them practise beyond their level of competence and do not deserve even the much lower remuneration they demand. Besides, a lot of unethical practices that doctors are accused of actually started with quacks and since doctors are competing in the same market as them, they are ultimately forced to adopt these malpractices.

You may think the services of your 'jhola-chhaap doctor' or 'Bengali doctor' (alternative names for quacks) are very reasonable but little do you know that they invented the art of keeping consultation fees low (sometimes nil) and earning almost exclusively through cuts from laboratories and hospitals, a practice that our doctors too are now seen indulging in.

Are Quacks Effective?

A large number of human illnesses are self-limiting and an equally large number will respond to OTC medicines that anyone could buy, quite legally, from any chemist shop. This works in the favour of our quacks. Furthermore, most of them have had some experience of working with doctors and know what doctors prescribe for common symptoms. This could be a chemist shop assistant who sees hundreds of prescriptions every day or a ward boy in a hospital or a physician's assistant. Then there is the recognized placebo effect, where a patient gets better simply because he thinks he is receiving the appropriate treatment. Such are the miraculous ways of the human body—a strong belief that one is receiving appropriate treatment is sometimes sufficient to bring about a cure.

Each such patient who is 'cured' at the hands of a quack then becomes a brand ambassador. Often, quacks use antibiotics and steroids to bring out quick symptomatic relief. This makes them look more effective. Not wanting to lose business, doctors have begun copying them. Similarly, infertility is a common problem but a large number of women will conceive naturally over a period of time. This is an ideal market for our quacks. I am not alluding to those religious gurus who rape women to 'cure' them of their husband's inability to inseminate them. I am talking about others who give out medicines to increase fertility among women or potency among men. The woman may conceive naturally and the quack gets the credit. Some quacks will carry out illegal abortions, even operations, without any training. Some will refer patients to hospitals or other specialists and claim commissions. Almost every quack prescribes and dispenses Allopathic medicines without any real knowledge. That they are sometimes successful cannot hide the fact that they remain hugely dangerous to the patients, and as we have seen above, though they may not charge much directly, the indirect cost to the patient (through loss of health and cost of unnecessary treatment) and society is much higher.

Two-Tier Health Care

It is true that India does not have the required number of doctors and the public sector, upon which the largely poor population depends completely, does not have the resources and the will to cope with the need. There can only be two ways to solve this problem—either train a large number of doctors and retain them with jobs in hospitals equipped to absorb them or dilute the level of qualification so as to allow anyone who so wishes to become a doctor. We know how the Indian government reacts when faced with such difficult choices. How did they reduce the number of poor in India? Not by creating more employment opportunities or by preventing exploitation of the poor by enforcing a respectable minimum living wage. They reduced the number of poor in India by further lowering the poverty line. In this context, it does not matter to our highly qualified bureaucrats and their political masters that the income which places the poor above this new imaginary line cannot even buy one meal for his family. Similarly, when it comes to health care, it does not matter who people see and whether that person can deliver worthwhile medical care. All the government can care about is that the person consulted is called a Registered Medical Practitioner. The government knows fully well that such RMPs pretend to be doctors and ultimately do everything that a regular doctor does, only without the requisite education and training. Yet, the government wants to bring all of a variety of quacks under this umbrella term and give them authentic licences. According to them, this is the only way to provide health care to the vast numbers of naïve, undiscerning poor living in Indian villages and urban slums. This is the best the poor deserve.

It is important, though, to examine the proffered logic. It is true that most patients present common symptoms like fever, cough, abdominal pain, headache, diarrhoea, etc. If somebody could just treat these conditions, we will need far fewer doctors. The argument is compelling. Create a second tier of professionals to treat these conditions and save the real doctors for real illnesses—a perfect solution to a difficult global problem. One wonders then why the rest of the world hasn't thought of it already and why they keep importing doctors and nurses from India. I think I may know why. Is it because the conditions described above are not medical conditions but the common symptoms of a very large number of medical conditions. It takes many years of education about the human body and its systems, knowledge about how various diseases affect it and how medicines work to be able to accurately diagnose and treat any patient. A patient with a cough, for example, could have one of a dozen medical conditions, as could a patient with abdominal pain. Medical science works based on doctors diagnosing these conditions with a degree of accuracy, backed up by diagnostic tests as and when necessary, and determination of the need for hospital treatment in a timely fashion. If we as a society genuinely believe that what a doctor learns through years of hard work and education can be replicated by somebody who has assisted him in his clinics for some time, then perhaps we should close down our medical colleges and save future generations of doctors the humiliation of working in a society that values them no more than a quack. Yes, doctors cannot provide adequate outpatient care in India and their standards of service are sometimes not vastly superior to that of quacks, but this is not because doctors don't know how to provide better health care. It is because quacks are driving down the standards. Doctors are competing with quacks. They cannot charge much more than a quack or spend much more time with a patient than a quack does or request diagnostic tests when a quack won't. By elevating quacks to the stature of doctors, we are bringing doctors down to the level of quacks.

Qualified doctors practising modern medicine can do a lot to set their own house in order but what certainly does not help their morale is having to rub shoulders with quacks, on a daily basis. Just like other professionals, doctors have a right to earn a dignified, honest living. This is made impossible when there are no proper jobs for the vast majority of them and they are forced to start their own private practices and compete with quacks for work. Qualified doctors are, at least on paper, regulated by professional bodies, the consumer courts and the justice system. Who is regulating quacks?

It is true that without quacks in our communities, a majority of poor and rural Indians will have nobody to go to. It is also sadly true that patients will continue to go to them for advice even once they know clearly what their qualifications are. After all, how many Indians, the middle class included, can afford private medical treatment? People take health-related advice from whoever can give it. Be it an assistant in a chemist shop, or a friend, or even a family member who has suffered from a similar illness. When we do this, we are doing it in full knowledge of the implications of our actions.

We know from our previous experiences with RMPs that any move to train quacks and bring them into the mainstream fold, in some sort of a paramedical role within our health care system, serves only to legitimize quacks and undermine doctors. If the government is really serious about the health of the poor, it needs to start thinking seriously about investing in health care and overcoming the barriers of corruption. If government primary health centres and district hospitals were fit to serve in the twenty-first century and manned by adequately paid doctors and nurses, in turn held accountable for lapses, we can have a health care system that we can be proud of. Giving licences to quacks to make a mockery of the life of the poor is not a solution to the problem; it is a recipe to entrench it deeper.

Pharmacy or Grocery Shop?

There is another huge problem that must be discussed in this context. In most countries, one cannot buy anything other than OTC medication from pharmacies. India is different; here, people can go to any pharmacy or medicine shop and buy any medicine they want. Buying and selling medicines in India works no differently from buying and selling groceries. You go with a list and you can buy any drug you like. On the face of it, we have rules. These rules prohibit selling of drugs other than OTC medications without the prescription of a qualified doctor. These rules also state that medicines should only be dispensed by a qualified pharmacist.

The reality, however, is different. I have not seen one pharmacy in India where shop assistants with no knowledge of pharmacy are not 'selling' medicines to any patient with or without a prescription. You give the list of what you want to buy to anybody in a shop, receive the goods and pay for it. It's that simple. Moreover, it does not matter if you do or do not have a doctor's prescription; you can buy whichever medicine you like anytime. If the government really wished to protect people from inappropriate use of medical drugs, restrictions on their buying and selling are indispensable. In this day and age, it is not impossible to ensure that every batch of scheduled drugs has a digital trail and that it cannot be bought or sold without prescription of a qualified doctor with his/her registration number (that can be easily verified on the MCI website) on it. In one stroke, this move will control all quackery, including self-quackery. Patients will then have to see qualified doctors for a prescription and quacks will not be able to buy medicines to dispense in coloured bottles and paper wrappings.

What works for Western societies may not always be applicable to India. I am not saying patients on long-term medication need a new prescription every month. I am not even saying that every medicine needs a prescription; we can come up with our own more inclusive list of OTC drugs that can be freely dispensed. All I am saying is that allowing people to prescribe and buy medicines freely is neither cheap nor safe. Patients are paying quacks and then spending money on medicines. What are they getting in return? Are they really getting a qualified medical opinion? Are they really spending money on a medicine they need? I'll go a step further. They might just wash this money down the drain with possibly better outcomes.

Analogies are always inaccurate, as they don't compare like to like. But I can't resist the temptation of offering one in this context. Say for example, we don't have enough resources to train all the pilots we need. Would giving flying licences to the large number of existing car drivers solve the problem?

The Quack Nurse

Though much ink has been spilled describing the impact of quacks on doctors, not a tear has been shed for the plight of qualified nurses in India. Apart from a traditional mind-set which does not accord them with the respect they deserve, the fact that almost anybody can be given a nurse's uniform or 'trained' to be a nurse by scores of private nursing schools means that many nurses see no viable option other than migrating to other countries to feel valued and earn a decent wage. Stories of untrained people working as ward boys or technicians or biomedical engineers also exist. In all areas of health care delivery, trained professionals are forced to work alongside untrained people, and though the trained ones have spent many years studying and are held accountable by various professional bodies and the machinery of law, the untrained professionals reap the benefits without any talent to show for the job or any investment of time or money.

This lies at the heart of mass migration of doctors and nurses out of India. The same people who struggle to obtain a decent job here are valued as respected health care staff in almost all parts of the world. Ultimately, India is losing out. We are training our doctors and nurses, only for them to migrate to other countries.

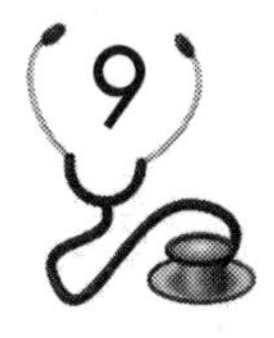

The Private Sector

Indian private hospitals treat patients as revenue generators.
—Indo Asian News Service, 25 Feb 2015

Indian corporate hospitals have destroyed the backbone of medical ethics.
—Dr Amit Ghose, Kolkata

Given the pathetic state our public sector health centres and hospitals are in, private health care is the only viable alternative available to a large section of the Indian population. According to various estimates, the private sector now serves roughly three quarters of the health care needs of our population. The private sector is also playing an increasingly dominant role in medical education now with private medical colleges outnumbering government medical colleges. Governments the world over never have enough money for all that they want to do. In India, bureaucracy and corruption result in only a tiny proportion of the allocated resources actually reaching the intended beneficiary. On the other hand, the private sector represents the free will of the people and is free from such hurdles and from any moral obligation to serve the people.

Private Nursing Homes and Hospitals

The Indian success story of the last two decades has been driven primarily by the private sector. We have proved beyond doubt that with a little support, Indians can become global leaders. Recent governments do deserve credit for facilitating and fostering the growth of private enterprise. But where governments in India have not done so well is in ensuring that the private sector works in an organized and regulated manner, synchronised with government machinery. This is nowhere more obvious than in the delivery of health care. The bulk of outpatient and inpatient health care in our country is provided by private clinics, nursing homes and hospitals, and these have mushroomed all over the country without proper planning or forethought. Yet there has been no effort to match supply with demand. Unregulated markets usually become dysfunctional and Indian health care is a perfect example of this phenomenon.

Though big corporate hospitals spring to mind foremost, they account for only a small percentage of private health care provided in India. Bulk of the care falls to independent freelance medical practitioners. Since there is no system in place to guarantee jobs offering adequate remuneration and infrastructure on completion of education, doctors have no choice but to open their own clinics and run them like businesses whilst competing with quacks. Those who are good at running the business then go on to open nursing homes and hospitals. Morality takes a back seat as professional ethics gives way to business practices.

Human beings are competitive by nature. We all want to be better than the guy next door. The more ambitious among us feel it more keenly, but almost everyone harbours within them at least a tiny seed of this urge to compete. 'Better', however, is a very broad word—we need to define in what ways we wish to better others. This is where our collective cherished values come in. Societies determine the domains of competition and individuals play their part. If society aspires to see individual doctors engage in more research, academics and honest, evidence-based practice, that is what doctors will aspire to achieve. And if societies fail to develop their own benchmarks of assessment, individuals will fall prey to human greed.

In my humble view, one of the most glaring collective failures of Indian society is our failure to establish ethical and progressive domains for competition. Consequently, professional roles have simply devolved into a race for money or power; there are no alternative benchmarks of respect and no other known way to prove one's dominance over others.

Infrastructure and Manpower

Though big hospitals have to follow many structural and professional norms, this does not apply to small clinics and nursing homes. As a result, doctors have opened a range of facilities for inpatient treatment depending on their financial strength. This translates to enhanced revenues, as patients needing inpatient treatment needn't be referred to any other facility. Moreover, doctors know a number of well-recognized tactics whereby they can charge uneducated, unsuspecting, helpless patients higher fees. I remember a doctor from a small town telling me many years ago that you can only charge Rs 10 for a consultation but if you give an injection, you can charge

Rs 100 and if you have a facility with a bed where you can administer intravenous fluids (commonly known as glucose), you can charge in hundreds.

It does not take long to figure out that in private Indian health care, profits depend on the size of the facility—bigger the facility, higher the profit. One can start with whatever one can manage; put in some beds and a nursing home is born. The next step is to have a high dependency unit or an Intensive Care Unit (ICU) and an Operating Theatre (OT). Buildings that house these facilities have variable standards, ranging from the most rudimentary and pathetic to those that are made to last, with all the adequate planning and forethought that should go into building a proper hospital.

Unsurprisingly, many of these facilities are not fit for purpose. Now my understanding of a nursing home is that of a facility placed somewhere between a home and a hospital, where you have nurses providing nursing care, hence the name. What we see in India are setups where people undergo almost all kinds of invasive medical treatments, including operations and intensive care. There is very little that one can't have done in a nursing home these days.

A large number of nursing homes with substandard facilities function like hospitals, completely inadequate for the purpose they ought to serve. Many don't have beds that can be called hospital beds. Oxygen is provided in cylinders and drips hang off worn-out metal stands. Many don't have in-house facilities to run basic blood tests and radiological investigations. Sometimes, there are ICUs without even a ventilator or an Intensivist (a doctor specializing in critical intensive care). God only knows who operates these ventilators. In such places, basic infection control and sanitation measures are lacking. Patient privacy is often out of question. The bottom line is that if the alternative state facilities weren't much worse, patients wouldn't go to these nursing homes.

Such nursing homes also carry out operations using crude and often outdated OTs and equipment. Anaesthetic equipment and machines are usually poorly maintained and the methods of sterilization of surgical instruments are open to challenge. In many such places that I have been to, I couldn't see any separation of hospital waste from ordinary waste, or basic fire precautions and other safety mechanisms in place.

I hope you get the picture. There simply is no restriction on a doctor who wishes to open a nursing home and he can do whatever he likes in such a facility. Authorities have squarely turned a blind eye to it all. For any hospital (or nursing home functioning like a hospital) to run effectively, a number of medical and paramedical staff are needed, including doctors available round the clock, trained nurses and technicians. In several cases, the doctor who owns the facility himself provides round-the-clock cover without any break in duty. Many such setups are run by doctor couples like a family-owned business. Doctors often live on the same premises and are on call throughout the day. Naturally, they can't work nonstop without any rest, which means patients getting admitted overnight are often at the mercy of nurses and ward boys or junior doctors with very little experience. In Western countries, doctors are governed by work hour directives and patients can legally challenge if they are being looked after by an overworked and tired doctor. These rules don't apply to India in general and such nursing homes in particular, where the same doctor is on call every day of the week. In these nursing homes, whether or not a doctor will come down to see you when you need them depends on your luck.

Moreover, the owners often work outside their areas of training and competence, and the support staff may not always be fit for purpose. Modern medicine is becoming increasingly complex and it is impossible for one doctor to provide adequate inpatient care to patients suffering from all kinds of ailments. We must differentiate here between inpatient care, where a patient needs to be admitted to a medical facility and outpatient care, where a patient is well enough to not need admission to a hospital. Trained General Practitioners (GPs) can provide early outpatient care for almost all illnesses. A GP is, however, specifically trained to identify signs and symptoms of serious illnesses which should prompt referral to a hospital. It is a different matter altogether that the majority of doctors in India who work as GPs or family doctors have not obtained any specialist training in general practice. What usually happens is that the doctor(s) owning these nursing homes tend to themselves treat almost any patient who walks through the door. When these doctors are truly out of their depth and are well aware that this is so (and it is rare that they are aware), they will call specialists to their facilities to seek their opinion, and sometimes, to perform operations. There is no shortage of people in Indian health care willing to provide such services on a freelance basis.

The fact that the facility is owned and run by the same doctors means it is open to regulatory abuse with no scope for external monitoring. Indeed, there is no transparency about what goes on within these premises. Patients here truly are at the mercy of God.

The Regulatory Vacuum

Private Indian health care delivery simply has no provisions for monitoring clinical outcomes and results of individual doctors. There is hardly any inbuilt accountability or external overseeing in the system. Mechanisms of auditing and clinical governance are largely non-existent.

There are islands of excellence, no doubt, but there are vast seas of incompetence and substandard medical care. The fatal combination of greed and incompetence in many cases amounts to the patient ultimately losing both money and health. Patients are admitted depending on whether the beds are going unused; tests are ordered not out of genuine need but to maximize revenue; unnecessary treatments are prescribed and patients are rarely involved in the decision-making.

Corporate Hospitals

Many senior doctors I have spoken to blame big private nursing homes and corporate hospitals for declining ethical standards in the medical profession. 'They have brought a business ethos into the profession, where revenue and profit are the only things that matter,' they point out.

Most of them have an army of marketing executives, whose sole job is to maintain a close relationship with doctors in the community. These executives are empowered to organize lavish lunches, give out expensive gifts and of course, arrange the commission for referring doctors.

There are lots of doctors out there looking to become health care tycoons. They want to build big hospitals and own hospital chains. This is only possible if they charge patients exorbitant sums of money. Often, a lower sum is quoted to start with, but the final bill is much higher with all the hidden charges that weren't revealed earlier. If the patient has an insurance policy, the doctor will make sure it is fully used.

Now, insurance fraud is seen in other countries too, but in India, the situation appears to be much worse. An insurance policy often is a guilt-free way for the doctor to rob the patient; it is a victimless crime. After all, what's wrong in extracting money from big insurance companies? Patients play their own part in such fraud. I am told some hide illnesses to buy an insurance policy to get free treatment. Of course, this translates to a higher premium for everyone and puts insurance beyond the means of even middle class families, but why should individuals care? Isn't it the government's responsibility? It is true that people who contribute the least to society complain the most about governments doing nothing.

The treatment you get in many hospitals depends on the doctor's estimate of your paying capacity. A doctor can keep you in hospital unnecessarily for days, give you one expensive medicine after another, put you on a ventilator, do an operation, or anything else he can think of to maximize your bills. As a patient, you have no means of knowing if any of this is strictly necessary. You cannot complain against anybody, and even if you could, to whom would you turn? You have a choice. You can go to a different doctor; many patients do take a second and a third opinion when they have time to plan ahead. However, what is the guarantee that the second doctor is going to be any better than the first? It is the responsibility of the government, and not the public, to ensure that doctors are adequately trained and regulated. To expect this from a government which can't even prevent hundreds of thousands of quacks from openly treating patients is nothing short of living in cloud cuckoo land.

Doctors themselves are at the mercy of hospitals. These hospitals have marketing machinery operating locally, regionally, nationally, and even internationally. As a doctor, affiliation to these institutions can radically transform your private practice and it is in your interest to be attached to one or more of them. Nursing homes and hospitals know how desperate doctors are. In these institutions, your continued attachment depends on how much business you can bring. It is understood that you will employ one or more of the recognized tactics, described elsewhere in this book, to maximize business for yourself and for the hospital. In fact, if you don't indulge in these practices, you risk earning the tag of 'too ethical' (as one doctor I know was labelled by a corporate hospital marketing executive) and hence not worth supporting or promoting.

Many hospitals give doctors revenue targets that they must achieve. Failure to do so could imperil their connection with the hospital. Imagine then what these doctors have to do to survive. I am not trying to justify any doctor ordering any unnecessary test, or recommending unnecessary hospital admission or treatment, or performing an unnecessary operation. I am trying to understand the rationale underlying this behaviour that has now become endemic in contemporary Indian medical practice. In many hospitals, doctors operate on a percentage basis. For example, as a doctor, you get 10 per cent of total patient bills. In this system of perverse incentives, it is in your direct interest then to maximize the patient's bills. Moreover, there is somebody in the hospital machinery closely monitoring the doctors. For example, somebody who can tell the bosses how many potential 'customers' you have been able to convince to have an operation; it does not matter if the patients did or did not really the procedure. They were sent to you by somebody for an operation, and so it was your job to perform one. If you do not, the GP (who had convinced the patient to come and see you) and the hospital marketing executive (the middleman) will not bring you further business.

The rules of the game are simple. As a doctor, you engage with the system and there is no end to where you can get; you bring ethics into it and the water gets a bit muddy. Doctors who are proficient at playing this game are promoted by the hospital through their marketing machinery, and those who are not are usually deemed unworthy of further investment. After all, marketing machinery is where these nursing homes and hospitals really have an upper hand. They have the required financial muscle and can afford to have teams of marketing executives. Most importantly, they are legally allowed to operate and advertise like businesses. Individual doctors, on the other hand, are bound by the code of conduct laid down by the MCI and are not allowed to advertise themselves. This is where the hypocrisy of our system is completely exposed. If you work for a hospital, they can advertise your services. They are only allowed to advertise their services without promoting specific doctors, yet I have come across newspaper advertisements where doctors' names were also mentioned. So there is a race to join big corporate hospitals. For hospitals, it is a win-win situation; they can pick and choose. Those who are popular, those who know how to attract business and those willing to engage with the system will be handpicked and nurtured. For the rest, a tag of mediocrity and a lifetime of struggle will define their future.

One understands the need for any business to be financially viable and essentially, these hospitals are businesses. Responsibility, in my opinion, must chiefly rest with the government and the regulators who have let the culture deteriorate. What will hospitals do if no doctor will refer patients to them irrespective of the quality of the services? What can hospitals do if quacks run half the industry? How can we expect corporate hospitals to share the results transparently when public sector hospitals and small private nursing homes operate with impunity and a complete lack of accountability? Corporate hospitals have had to learn how to attract business and survive and I don't for a moment believe it is entirely their fault. These hospitals add enormous value to health care delivery. Without them, millions of people will have no viable service for their health care needs, and thousands of doctors and nurses no jobs.

Service to Public

Many private hospitals are built on public land provided by the government at a subsidized rate. They can avail of many benefits simply because they provide health care. For example, import duty reduction on many medical items. Such benefits are not available to other industries. When these institutions want favours from the government, they are quick to flash the health care tag but if anyone brings up the issue of giving back to society, they want to be treated like businesses. Many of these institutions are supposed to offer free beds for the poor. But these beds often go unused, as mechanisms to avail of them are not transparent. At the same time, there is no sign of any government machinery that could hold them to their side of the bargain. As a result, this has become a profitable industry. The government provides the land, doctors and nurses with nowhere else to work are forced to work for them on their terms, and with our public health care in a shambles, patients are only too grateful to have a local hospital they can go to.

The Way Out

It is not impossible to change the outlook of health care in India, especially if our policy makers and politicians showed some will. No one is suggesting that it is going to be easy but the alternative is chaos. We have a choice, but not for too long.

Why are we allowing these institutions to come up all over the country without any planning or forethought? Why are we allowing nursing homes and hospitals to treat patients so flippantly? Why don't we ask them to furnish evidence to vouch for their capability to treat the conditions and diseases they claim to treat? Why can't we develop some sort of mechanism to monitor results of doctors and hospitals? Why do we not start developing systems where every doctor and nurse graduating from medical colleges has a job to go to that pays them a decent wage comparable to others in society. These jobs don't have to be in the government sector only. I agree that our government, as in many other countries, does not have the resources to cater to all the people under its aegis, but why can't it try to develop an inclusive framework wherein both the public and the private sector can set up services to provide seamless health care to people.

It is inconceivable that a nursing home owned by an orthopaedic surgeon can offer treatment for all kinds of medical conditions. Can we not ask nursing homes to clearly list the diseases they can treat properly? Such a list should be clearly displayed on the premises. It is also not impossible to ask these places to have designated doctors who are competent in providing care for these 'listed' medical conditions, available round the clock. Once it is known what services a nursing home wants to offer, it is also possible to figure out what all will be required for it to function smoothly and the authorities can ensure that continued operational licences are only given out if all infrastructure and human resource requirements are met. These facilities should be required to audit their key figures on a periodic basis. Another key step would be to carry out periodic case reviews and external checks to ensure appropriate medical standards are being met.

One of the biggest problems with organization of private health care in India is that there is no effort to match supply to demand. This has meant that there are areas where there are too many nursing homes and hospitals competing for too few patients who can afford their services and there are other areas where patients, even those who are willing to pay, simply have nowhere to go. There is no easy solution to this problem as it can only be effectively tackled by large-scale development of rural India. But concentrating all services in some towns and cities is not the answer either. I think it would be perfectly reasonable to cap the numbers of doctors, specialists and inpatient beds in any given geographical area. Imposing an upper limit this way will spread the manpower and services out into unserved areas. To further encourage such enterprise in rural areas, the government could pitch in with land for the premises and tax-free periods to improve sustainability. Governments have huge powers at their disposal. If these powers were used to incentivize development of rural health care, private practitioners would flock there. The alternative is that we let them build more and more hospitals in already over-served big cities and kill each other (and the medical profession) with their unethical practices.

Private Medical Colleges

We Indians have the habit of aiming too high and then falling short. This is best exemplified in our claims at moral values. Take the case of private education. There is nothing wrong with the underlying principle that we seem to have espoused. Education is the right of every child, not the exclusive privilege of those who can afford to pay exorbitant fees. One cannot really argue against education not being allowed to run like a business either. After all, just like we believe medicine is a noble profession and doctors should not be bothered about making money, teaching should be for saints. These principles may have once been a guiding force of life in our country, but that was last done successfully some 2,000 years ago. The reality of contemporary India is different; teachers and doctors need to earn a livelihood. Respect in society largely follows money, and not the attitude to serve. And institutions need to be financially viable to be able to continue and to prosper.

It is not easy to set up a medical college in India. Let us look at some of the provisions of the 'Establishment of Medical College Regulations' of 1999. First of all, a college can only be opened by the government or under the umbrella of a society, a charitable trust, or an autonomous body promoted by the government. Without going into the legal details, it basically means that you cannot expect to run it like a business and must have support from the government. Yet, you must have 25 acres of land and a 300-bedded (this part has since been amended a bit) hospital with the requisite infrastructure. It doesn't end there. The government also wants private medical colleges to take in students through a common entrance test, reserve a large number of seats for government-sponsored candidates, and have control over the fees they can charge from students.

Since we have effectively excluded businesses from setting up medical colleges and with all the rules and regulations made the whole exercise financially non-viable, the only people interested are those who know how to play the system. No doubt, many of these colleges have been set up and are being run by genuine charitable trusts but many others have been set up by people with no interest in social causes. Aspiration to the highest ideals has only meant that it is impossible to set up a private medical college without political patronage. The desire to over-regulate has only resulted in more black money exchanging hands in the form of capitation fees, a market estimated to run into thousands of crores.

There is nothing wrong with governments setting ground rules that reflect the aspirations of the people. But it is also important that these rules are practical and possible to implement. Currently, we have many more rules than our regulator or government can dream of enforcing. Not only that, our government responds to departures from current rules with even more rules, instead of reinforcing regulating mechanisms. A rule is only as robust as the ability to enforce and regulate it. One day our masters will wake up to this reality.

India needs more doctors and more jobs for doctors. Private medical colleges and their hospitals could prove to be a boon for our health care system if only the government showed some vision and flexibility. Money is required to run world-class hospitals and medical colleges. Since the government doesn't have enough to support its own institutions, it couldn't even dream of supporting the private sector. The present day governmental philosophy of interfering with everything defies the very purpose of free enterprise. I agree that it is the government's duty to ensure social justice but this needs to be achieved through strengthening its own institutions, enabling them and building more of them, rather than obstructing the autonomy of private institutions. All that the government needs to do is to ensure that these medical colleges produce able professionals, without involving itself much in the process. If the MCI simply vouched for the infrastructure and faculty requirements being met and for the end result being an adequately trained doctor (ratified by a national exit examination), we would have a well-functioning system.

It should not concern the government too much how these private institutions select students and how much they charge them. It is a market out there and private medical colleges compete with institutions not just within the country but also abroad to attract the best students, and they must be allowed to do so. I am not saying markets will always function efficiently and effectively. I am saying governments should not *run* the market, only *regulate* them.

If these institutions are financially viable, they will be able to attract world-class faculty and retain them, develop research facilities to provide a stimulating environment, and aspire to become global benchmarks. The current scenario is exactly the opposite though. The government decides who establishes these colleges and what sort of students they enrol. It even wants to decide the fees charged. Then the government blames these colleges when they have no money to actually run a hospital or recruit faculty and produce professionals who have not gone through a robust process of assessment. Too much regulation in India is the root cause of pervasive corruption and lawlessness.

The revenue obtained legally from NRI students and illegally from the management quota subsidizes the education of government quota students in private medical colleges. It is not impossible to understand why ordinary students coming through government quota and their parents welcome this subsidization. Individuals always want the best for themselves, but societies have to think of the collective good. If the end result is that our private medical colleges become non-viable, have no resources to recruit any faculty, and cannot actually give satisfactory education and training to any student, we are betraying not just those who paid their way into these institutions but also those who came through the government quota. Let us not forget that it is not just these doctors we are failing, but also millions of patients these ill-trained doctors will see over a lifetime.

I come from a very middle-class family myself and if I hadn't been lucky enough to be selected to a government medical college, I don't think my parents would have had the resources to be able to send me to a private medical college. Children growing up in families with limited resources must be able to obtain higher education in order to break the social ceiling. It is important that children can aspire to a better life than their parents and can access opportunities to do so. Hence, it is important that alongside steps to empower our government and private medical colleges, we also take steps to support students from disadvantaged backgrounds. Such support mechanisms don't have to undermine the financial viability of private medical colleges. Western countries use student loans and bursaries for these purposes. So far India has lagged behind in developing such mechanisms. It is in the interest of any institution to be able to attract the best students. If private medical colleges are financially successful, they will want to create scholarships for the best students who can't otherwise afford to study on their campuses. Student loans are going to prove much trickier to develop at a mass level for a country like India but it is not beyond the means of the government of the day to help develop financial products that allow very low interest rates and delayed repayment for students. Finally, the philanthropic sector could also help in supporting students with limited means.

Essentially, what I am saying is that private medical colleges need to be allowed complete freedom to set their fee structure and not be burdened with too many quotas. I would want to go further and apply the same to our government medical colleges. The latter operate from dilapidated buildings with poor infrastructure and largely face the same challenges in retaining high quality faculty and developing a research environment that private medical colleges do. Bureaucratic control and lack of financial independence has hindered the progress for our government medical colleges and hospitals. Viability of these institutions and interests of poorer students don't have to be mutually exclusive. If our colleges and universities can't charge students a fair fee, they can't invest in infrastructure and recruit world-class facility. As a result, they lag behind in research and academic output, which means they cannot attract big research grants. Ultimately, everybody loses—the institutions, the public, the faculty, and certainly the students. A different approach could be giving our government institutions complete autonomy in running their affairs. If they can charge a fair fee, decide remunerations for their faculty and generate their own revenue, they may, just like their private counterparts, actually have the resources to develop means-tested bursaries, scholarships and student loans for those who need such support.

Another issue that needs to be addressed when it comes to running our educational institutions is the intake of students. This has been hugely controversial in the recent past with a plan to develop a National Eligibility Entrance Test (NEET) suggested by the MCI and now upheld by the Supreme Court of India. Amid strong reservations expressed by several states against conducting the NEET, the NDA government in May 2016 paved the way for an ordinance to keep state governments' exams out of the ambit of the common test. President Pranab Mukherjee passed the ordinance on 24 May 2016. In addition to the huge problem of redefining the target for hundreds of thousands of students who may already have prepared for a different examination at virtually no notice at all, mandating all institutions in the country to use only one score will have its own implications.

I must make it clear here that the devil will lie in details and it remains to be seen if institutions would be allowed to use some other criteria to supplement the scores of this test for their intake. Furthermore, any examination only assesses the education and knowledge students have obtained in the preceding years. Numerous state examinations take care of the varied background of their students. It remains to be seen how NEET will account for it. Many states see it as an infringement on their rights and a test that they believe will put students pursuing education in state systems at a disadvantage compared to those with for example the Central Board of Secondary Education (CBSE). There are other problems. Many private and premier government institutions have opposed this move, as they want some control over who can access their resources. World-class educational institutions need to be able to continue to attract the best students to retain their place in a competitive academic environment. Moreover, in a country, where papers are often leaked, can the best institutions really be asked to rely solely on the results of a national test to decide their intake? It is also worth recognizing that assessment of merit has more dimensions than what a simple multiple choice question paper can assess.

In an ideal world, we could have a national test rolled out, after adequate warning to the states and the students, that gives out scores and students then apply to a number of institutions with such a score. If individual medical colleges then want to conduct further brief tests or interviews, I cannot see any reasonable objection to it as long as the processes are fair, transparent and subject to external scrutiny. And, monitoring these processes is where the government needs to concentrate its efforts.

It is not possible for the government to control everything and the more it wants to control, the less it actually can. The Indian government needs to develop methods of liberating public institutions from the shackles of bureaucracy and empowering private ones. Only then will it be able to do its own job properly, which is to monitor and regulate the system. There has been massive population explosion and extension of the human lifespan over the past few centuries. As a direct consequence, the role of governments has changed. In modern societies, it is to enable, empower and monitor people, institutions and markets, not control them.

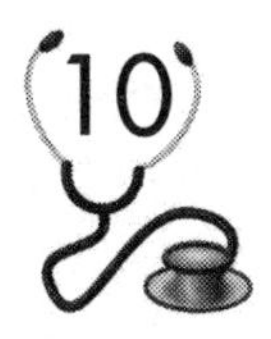

The Public Sector

Overall, the nation's vast, government-run health system can be a dangerous place. Hospitals are decades out-of-date, short-staffed and filthy. Patients frequently sleep two to a bed.

—The *Wall Street Journal*, 30 July 2011

Almost 4 million BPL (Below Poverty Line) households had to bribe hospital staff to get services like getting admission in the hospital, getting a bed, diagnostic services and getting an OPD card. The total amount of bribe paid to the hospital staff/official by the poor in the last one year is estimated to be Rs 870 million. Nearly 1 million households were denied hospital services simply because they either refused to offer bribes or could not afford that kind of money to pay the hospital staff/official.

—Transparency International India, 27 June 2008

Even (going) by standards in India, where corruption is routine, the scale of the scam in the central state of Madhya Pradesh is mind-boggling. Police say that since 2007, tens of thousands of students and job aspirants have paid hefty bribes to middlemen, bureaucrats and politicians to rig results for medical schools and government jobs.

—The *Washington Post*, 5 July 2015

Modern health care is expensive and beyond the reach of the common man. Societies have developed their own mechanisms to fund it but it is a fact that without state support, the poor in any society will have no health care. With a large proportion of population living in extreme poverty, India has no choice but to develop an effective, efficient, answerable and responsive public health care system. Without it, hundreds of millions of people will continue to have no reasonable choice when ill.

Today's India is full of paradoxes. A country struggling to meet even the most basic health care needs of a majority of its population is also one of the biggest hubs of medical tourism. On one hand, we have a large number of private doctors and hospitals in desperate need of patients. On the other, we have a much larger patient pool, no doctor or hospital wants to look at. A country with an acute shortage of doctors and nurses is also the world's biggest exporter of medical manpower. We are probably one of the most religious-minded people in the world but also the most heartless when it comes to looking after the poor and the vulnerable. As a people, we constantly claim to live by high ideals and principles, yet we live in one of the most corrupt societies of this world. It surprises the world to see a country where dogs share beds with patients in a hospital can coexist with one of the most active space programmes known to mankind. It doesn't surprise Indians though. We grow up with these contradictions all around us.

Lack of accountability is the biggest problem of the Indian public systems. Rarely is any babu ever asked to explain his actions or lack thereof. Absence of adequate punitive measures in the system is probably the single most important contributory reason behind this scenario. Lack of bureaucratic autonomy and too much political control means that our senior civil servants do not believe they are answerable to the public. How can you be held responsible for somebody else's decisions? Politicians, on the other hand, rarely last more than five years and I am talking about the lucky ones. Brave bureaucrats can wage a war against corrupt and crime-friendly politicians, but it will be a war involving significant risk and sacrifice. I believe it is wrong to ask that of an ordinary civil servant who just wants to do a good job and earn a decent living, without carrying the burden of a battle on his shoulders. Such bravery is only expected of soldiers in India and one does wonder what will become of this country if our defence forces also started behaving like our bureaucracy. One also wonders what lessons can be learnt from the systems that regulate our defence establishments and whether they can be extrapolated to cover our civil services.

Investment

Good employers know that hiring good candidates is not enough. They need to be enabled and empowered to take the right decisions and then resourced to implement these decisions. Only then can they be held accountable and responsible. In Indian health care, and in public sector systems generally, these basic qualities that define a good employer are invisible. We have a system that aims at delivering too much with too little and then expectedly falls far short, without any provisions to review the responsibility or learn lessons. Such failures are a hallmark of our public sector planning, the end result being a system that does not work for the public it claims to serve and demoralizes the extremely talented but powerless civil service work force.

Take the case of Primary Health Centres (PHCs) for example. Every PHC is supposed to serve a defined rural area. According to the government's own documents: 'A typical Primary Health Centre covers a population of 20,000 in hilly, tribal, or difficult areas and 30,000 in plain areas with 4–6 indoor/observation beds. It acts as a referral unit for 6 sub-centres and refers out cases to CHCs (Community Health Centres, 30-bedded hospitals) and higher order public hospitals located at sub-district and district level.' As of September 2014, India had 25,020 PHCs. If, based on the 2011 census, one were to simply divide India's population by the number of PHCs, we would see that each PHC looks after approximately 48,400 people. If you add to that the likely variation in population density, you can rest assured that some PHCs look after twice as many people as they are meant to.

A PHC is supposed to be staffed by fifteen to eighteen people with at least one doctor and a range of other staff. Owing to difficulties in recruiting doctors to these PHCs, the government is increasingly looking at AYUSH (Ayurveda, Yoga and Naturopathy, Unani, Siddha and Homeopathy) practitioners to meet the demand. Typically, a PHC works on a budget of around 12–15 lakhs, the majority of which is spent on paying out salaries. They are supposed to provide a range of preventive, emergency and elective care to the population they serve using the available resources. Now, I don't know if we all live in the real world, because our policy makers clearly don't. If they did, they couldn't have failed to notice that a typical engineering graduate, who hasn't been lucky enough to land a job abroad, will earn anywhere between Rs 50,000 to 1,00,000 per year at the very least, in India. And a good middle-level employee in any private organization or a private doctor working independently in any of our towns and cities will expect to earn at least Rs 1–2 lakh per month to be able to pay a mortgage, afford a car, send his children to school, look after his parents, pay all the bills (and the bribes), the insurance premiums, and of course, save for the future. This is not luxurious living but the basic minimum standard a middle-class professional aspires to achieve sooner or later in life.

We want to run a PHC at Rs 10–12 lakh a year and then blame doctors for not wanting to work there. Which doctor in his right mind would sacrifice his dreams to live a rural life working for the salaries offered here, with no resources to practise scientific evidence-based medicine? Have you have been to any Indian village in the recent past? I have, and I can assure you that all the developments of the last two decades have not spread more than 10 kms beyond Gurgaon (taking National Capital Region, the NCR, for example). Working in Indian villages, given the condition they are in currently, can only be described as 'social service' or 'sacrifice'. It is not a job that anybody will aspire to. Yes, I might do it for a few years, like people who go to the Gulf, if I knew I would get paid enough to be able to secure the future of my family. The point I am making is that health care is not cheap and if the government wants doctors to work in villages, it has to pay them competitive wages in line with what others are earning elsewhere in the country and abroad. Otherwise, doctors will continue to move to bigger cities and foreign countries.

If we reward doctors with appropriate remuneration and state-of-the-art working facilities, we would have the adequate leverage to ask them to deliver their side of the bargain or they risk their job. The present day scenario, where nobody wants the job in the first place, doesn't really leave us in any position to negotiate. This means that the government will be hard pressed to continue driving down overall standards. Employing quacks (AYUSH practitioners are not doctors recognized by the Indian Medical Regulations of 2002 and as such not governed by those principles) as doctors is only the first detrimental step.

The Indian government has set aside Rs 29,143 crores for education, health and broadcasting for the year 2015–16. If we were to spend this entire budget on 25,020 PHCs alone, we would be spending Rs 1.16 crore per PHC every year. Even if every single paisa were actually spent on resourcing and staffing PHCs, without any loss due to corruption or inefficiency, there would be barely enough money to man and manage a modern PHC. Now maths was never my strong point, but I hope I have been able to give you an idea of the scale of the problem at hand and how much investment is needed to make a visible difference.

According to the latest World Bank statistics, India spends USD 61 per person on health compared to USD 3,647 spent by the UK and USD 8,895 by the Americans. In GDP terms, we spend 4 per cent of our GDP on health care compared to 9.4 per cent by the UK and 17.9 per cent by the US. These numbers include both public and private spend. If you were to look at public spending alone, the Indian government spends a mere 1.3 per cent of its GDP on health compared to 7.8 per cent by the UK and 8.3 per cent by the US. So what we have here is not just a poor country, which sadly India is, but a poor country where the government places health very low on its rung of priorities. The problem does not end there. India is also one of the most corrupt countries (ranked last year by Transparency International at number 85 out of 175 countries), which means that even the money allocated does not reach the beneficiary. Finally, needless to mention, we have some real visionaries as politicians who can't think beyond the next general elections and some very talented bureaucrats who have little freedom to challenge their political masters. If the forefathers of our constitution had intended for us to live in a democracy where politicians and bureaucrats kept a check on each other, sadly, that has not materialized. Our bureaucracy is impotent against politicians not because there aren't enough provisions in the rulebooks for fair balance, but because our politicians have systematically weakened the law and order machinery and strengthened themselves by joining hands with criminals.

Super Specialty Medical College Hospitals

At the other end of the available range of public sector health facilities are super specialty government medical colleges located in big cities. These hospitals not only provide complex treatments for a range of medical conditions but also train future generations of doctors and nurses. As of 17 August 2015, according to the MCI website, out of a total of 409 medical colleges with a total of 49,940 undergraduate seats, 191 are government owned and account for 25,580 seats. Government medical colleges also provide the bulk of postgraduate medical training in India. It is worth examining separately the patient care and education function of these institutions.

Given how expensive private hospitals are, the poor in this country face a stark choice between getting some treatment or none at all. It is only the sheer desperation of an illness that drags them to government hospitals. These are not places where they will be treated with respect, compassion, care, or even competence. Patient care here is handed out as a favour and a patient must politely and gracefully accept what is given. Questioning any doctor is unthinkable and mechanisms to lodge complaints against doctors and nurses are impossible to access even in places where such mechanisms do exist. If it is true that the environment in which health care is delivered—the hospital building, the bed, the toilets, the lights, the temperature, the food itself—have a lot to do with the healing process, I can guarantee these principles do not really apply to Indian government hospitals. Here, perfectly normal people will become sick and those with a fragile constitution will not be able to pass through a ward without vomiting out their last meal. One can expect to share the ward with a variety of stray animals. Touts and all kinds of sexual predators freely roam around in the guise of hospital staff, and doctors can be seen shouting at or slapping patients.

Locating the right department in the midst of a scattered clutter of buildings and structures is not easy. Even hospital staff don't usually know where a particular department is.

Indeed, when faced with a deluge of patients, triaging can be a difficult business. Triaging is exactly what you need to do when dealing with enormous demand for a limited resource. You could allocate the resource on a first come first serve basis. You could distribute it on the basis of clinical need. You could even argue that no sick patient will be turned away and public sector hospitals just have to learn to work with each other and with the private sector to look after at least those who need urgent inpatient hospital care. But the ground reality shows an absence of any such logically driven operating mechanism. In an environment characterized by an almost complete lack of transparency and accountability, bribery and nepotism, rather than any systematic policy, decide whether or not a hospital bed can be found. A patient who has neither money nor influence (which is usually why he would have gone to a government hospital in the first place), must brace himself for long frustrating waits as he is passed on from one hospital to the other. It is not as if there are ambulances available to take the patient from one hospital to another; he will have to manage in a taxi, auto, bus or any other vehicle he can find. If the patient dies in transit, let me disillusion you by telling that the system could not care less.

Medical Education and Postgraduate Training

Junior, in-training, newly graduated doctors deliver bulk of the care in government medical college hospitals. Most junior doctors with their eyes on the next competitive examination are desperate to somehow finish the work. Such is the nature of Indian health care and society—even young doctors, just starting out, become immune to all the moving influences in no time. These are young impressionable people who need to be trained to think critically and compassionately. They need to be exposed to systematic algorithmic thought that is now a vital part of modern medicine; they must be monitored and supervised, until they blossom into caring, competent clinicians. In the absence of effective role models, these doctors grow up learning and believing that money is everything and the lives of the poor don't matter.

Mistakes are bound to happen when they work thus with no support and little supervision—some hit the news, but the majority never come to surface. Before you misconstrue what I am saying, not for a moment do I believe that the fault lies with the young doctors. The fault lies with our machinery, which cannot ensure that all doctors are actually adequately educated before they get their degrees, which fails to give them adequate support when they start out, and finally, fails to hold them accountable for negligence and personal failure.

In many places, junior doctors work insane hours in pathetic conditions. In others, they work for half the time they are meant to, while essential patient care is delegated to ward boys and nurses. Mechanisms to ensure structured, guaranteed training are scarce, the remuneration unfit for a doctor, and job satisfaction is very low. In interventional specialties, new doctors are truly at the mercy of their seniors as they cannot really learn the steps unless somebody properly shows them how to do things and takes them through the steps a few times. But why would a senior do this when, in his early days, he had to learn it all by himself? So the end result often is a professional with a specialist degree, but not the requisite ability, who is then let loose in the society to learn and to earn. Such a professional will need patients to achieve both goals and he will be competing with those already established in the field. What is he likely to do to secure a regular flow of patients?

Currently, we have a number of government and private medical and nursing colleges churning out doctors and nurses based on a curriculum that rarely changes fast enough to reflect the changing needs of patients. Very few of these institutions have academic recognition in the global community and opportunities for research and academic development are largely non-existent. Moreover, merely obtaining medical qualifications does not equip doctors with all the necessary skills they will need in their practice ahead. Hence, it is generally mandatory in most countries that doctors work as a trainee or in supervised roles for a number of years before being allowed to make independent decisions. Unfortunately, this is not the case in India, especially when it comes to general practice or primary care.

Faculty in Medical Colleges and Hospitals

Government medical college faculty are probably one of the most significant building blocks in the edifice of Indian health care. They have a dual responsibility—to train the future generations and to look after the health of the poorest in society. One would suspect that there would be a huge clamour for such jobs with fierce competition amongst doctors for the honour and the recognition that likely accompanies such positions. But that is not the case for most medical colleges in India and very few doctors actually aspire to these jobs. Academic jobs are sought after all over the world, then why not in India? To understand this, we will have to understand the typical life of a faculty member in these institutions.

First of all, appointments in these institutions usually take place through state health departments and are based on an archaic system where doctors, like other government employees, are continually transferred from one place to another. It is not my job to examine this system for the rest of society but I do strongly believe this method does not work for doctors. No specialist in his right mind will take up this job if part of the deal is to spend years in an ill-equipped Community Health Centre or District General Hospital. There are some central government run or independent institutes where you can be appointed for life. Understandably, these institutions perform better and usually have no difficulty in recruiting and retaining world-class faculty. It was in the interest of the foreign powers that governed India in the past to weaken the bureaucracy through a number of systematic mechanisms; the ability to transfer senior bureaucrats or officials to dead-end jobs at will is one such. Only those who engaged with the system were given 'lucrative' jobs in big cities; the rest were sent to rot until retirement in remote villages. These mechanisms are no longer necessary or relevant in independent India.

Academic jobs are only going to become attractive if the culture and environment is conducive to academic work. It is not easy to set up research units and it is beyond the means of underfunded Indian educational establishments to even dream of it. Western educational institutions are independent enough to raise finances over and above what the state offers them. They can raise money from agencies that fund research, from international students, and from their alumni network. Researchers are recruited based on their ability to engage with the recognized systems. Those who can publish and attract grants are made professors. Talent is recruited from all over the world and universities decide for themselves whom they take on board. Now contrast this with Indian universities and educational establishments. Usually, they can't control who works with them as faculty and what sort of students they take in. They have no freedom to manage their own finances. They can't raise any money independently. Their alumni happily donate millions of dollars to Western institutions, where they may have pursued only a fraction of their total education, but can't donate anything to Indian institutions even if they want to, as mechanisms to accept such donations do not exist.

It is a vicious circle. Our institutions have no money to attract the best professors or offer scholarships to the best students from around the world. They have no incentive to go to other developing and even developed countries (something that our private hospitals have done successfully with the onset of medical tourism) to attract students. People in charge are appointed by ministers or senior bureaucrats and their jobs do not depend on the performance of the institution. There are no benchmarks or systems to measure anybody's performance as deans, directors, chairmen, superintendents and principals come and go.

We need to pay competitive salaries to recruit and retain world-class talent. Mass exodus of talented work force from India is driven partly by the lure of living in a more organized society under the rule of law, but principally, it follows money. Indian doctors and engineers migrate to USA, UK, Canada, Australia and the Middle East because there they are paid more. We have someday got to wake up and realize that these countries are not stupid to give Indians jobs when their own employment figures are not 100 per cent. They are keen to attract talent because every such truly talented person spurs the economy onward and opens up jobs for many more. Not having money to recruit talent is a self-fulfilling prophecy and politicians of the day must break this vicious cycle if India wishes to regain some of her old glory.

In this globalized world, manpower is simply a commodity that follows market dynamics. There is a universal shortage of qualified health care professionals who, understandably, want to work in places that pay well, offer opportunities for further training and career growth, and enable a better quality life. For these benefits, people will move thousands of miles away from their families, and even accept discrimination. Any analysis of the migration of medical workforce out of India will be incomplete without attempting to understand the psychology of a nurse who is prepared to move to Saudi Arabia. In that country, she will most certainly face significant language issues, various forms of discrimination, often ridicule, and will have little freedom to move around on her own. The Saudis make their own laws and they are certainly not forcing anybody to come and work for them. Moreover, Saudi Arabia is not the only place where Indian nurses go.

The point I am trying to make here is that to achieve something better for themselves and their families, human beings will often go to great lengths. Doctors and nurses from India (including me), who work in the UK, sometimes face issues of a different kind at the hands of colleagues who simply presume that darker skin and accented English imply lack of intellect. There is even suggestion of systematic intolerance and lack of opportunities for leadership positions that work against overseas doctors. Many senior clinicians and managers in the National Health Service believe that Indian doctors should just do their routine work, and not aspire to higher positions. The ultimate truth of life is that you can only rise to your full potential in your own society. That many Indian doctors overcome all these challenges and break the barriers to excel even in countries like the UK and the US is only an indication of their sheer grit and determination.

It is undisputed that the faculty in Indian medical colleges and hospitals are underpaid. Wages are approximately a quarter of what private practitioners will eventually earn or what they would earn in a Western country. Yet we expect them to feel motivated to serve the poor for the rest of their life. It is not surprising then that they resort to private practice to supplement the income, coerce patients into going to their private clinics, or even accept bribes for the work they are being paid to do. What can we really do about this? It is not as if there is a huge pool of high quality doctors desperately clamouring for these underpaid jobs in substandard facilities.

Doctors are only one of a number of groups of people who need to work collaboratively to deliver effective health care. A doctor needs an array of support staff and efficient management to do his job. Just to give you a rough idea, senior doctors account for no more than 10 per cent of the total number of employees in any hospital, and doctors in total account for no more than a quarter. Doctors cannot do their job if the managers, the porters, the nurses and others will not. In public sector Indian hospitals, nobody can be challenged on grounds of poor competence or shoddy work. There are powerful unions in place and the backlash can be severe. The balance between worker rights and worker responsibility is periodically lost in a society where no one has any faith in law enforcement and people often take matters into their own hands. The work culture in public sector establishments in India is generally marked by its absence. Hospitals are no exception.

Faculty are expected to educate and train students but what is the guarantee that they are being given trainable candidates? Excessive reservation without any minimum benchmarks and corruption in entry into medical colleges has meant that many students simply do not have the talent necessary to absorb medical education. Moreover, when the faculty themselves are struggling with a lack of facilities, how are they going to teach students about the latest medical advances. It is neither possible to practise nor teach evidence-based modern medicine in a majority of Indian public hospitals. Faculty here are being forced to practise the medicine of the 1950s in an ill-funded, ill-resourced system at the mercy of bureaucrats who don't understand what doctors have to go through on a daily basis.

The Money

As we saw above, with our current budgetary allocation, even if we spent the entire amount on PHCs alone, it would still not address even this one area of public health care in our country. Then what should we do with the rest of public health care needs? The answer is rather simple. To run a modern, efficient health care system, we need to invest more in it. Governments keep stating that they want to increase funding to 2.0–2.5 per cent of the GDP from the present levels of 1.0–1.3 per cent, but this claim is without any real desire backing it. I would argue that even these proposed numbers would be insufficient and we should be thinking 5 per cent. We need some significant upfront investment in our hospitals and health centres that have been running underfunded for decades, if we wish to really bring them to the level our population deserves. Developed economies spend between 6–8 per cent of their GDP on health, and for good reason. The health of the people of a nation determines a lot of other things in society. An unhealthy society cannot progress.

Emergency Ambulance and Triaging Service

One of the most glaring deficiencies of our health care system is a complete lack of organized, coordinated emergency services. With some investment, is it really impossible to create a National Ambulance Service? This could then be used to create a massive database of regional hospitals and beds. Ambulance crew could take patients to a hospital with beds available and once public sector hospitals are full, we could then use private sector hospitals beds. In fact, I would go a step further and suggest that this is what the government should actively seek from the private sector. In lieu of subsidized land, reduction on duties and tax breaks, these hospitals provide a number of beds for free/subsidized emergency care for patients. Currently, such a mechanism does exist but the public cannot fully avail it, as private hospitals don't make it easy for patients to access these beds. Such an ambulance service will not be easy or cheap to develop but it is certainly not beyond the will of a nation. It is particularly shameful given the fact that every other country worth its name has a functioning ambulance service.

Standardize Education and Training

Not only do we need adequate national entry and exit benchmarks for doctors, things that I have talked about elsewhere in this book, but we also need to ensure every graduating doctor has an opportunity for further training at a reasonable salary. In fact, we should make it mandatory. Medical education does not and cannot prepare one for all the challenges that lie ahead. Doctors need further training for a number of years to be able to put to practical use the knowledge they have gained. There is no reason why willing corporate hospitals and private primary care doctors could not be roped in to develop a training programme for every single medical graduate in the country who wants further training.

Finally, to round off on the subject, I wish to acknowledge that despite all its failures, the Indian public health care system does of course heal some sick. You may not have a penny in your pocket and your clothes might stink, but you could still walk into any government clinic or hospital and get some medical attention. Yes, the care available is not extremely sophisticated, it is not delivered by overly polite people, and may be substandard a lot of the time, but it *does* exist and it *is* administered. To those in this country who constantly criticize government doctors and nurses, I challenge them to try and spend one full day in these facilities before reaching any judgement. It is only befitting that a commentary on the state of our government-owned health care facilities also owes a heartfelt tribute to the sheer strength of character of the doctors and nurses who dedicate their lives to working in these institutions. They deserve to be accorded a stature no less than that conferred on those who stand at our country's borders, the only difference being the colour of their uniform. As always, the faults are all systemic, which is something these individuals are completely powerless against.

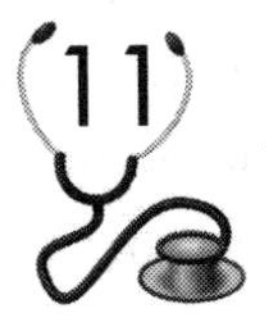

The Regulator

The private sector in India is represented by five star hospitals. Their services need to be regulated.

—World Health Organization

For a long time, the Medical Council of India has been a big source of corruption...instead of strengthening the components of medical education, it has weakened it.

—Dr Harsh Vardhan, Union Health Minister, June 2014

Around the world, societies have developed a number of regulators in different walks of life to guide human effort and action. It is these regulators that make it possible to monitor and control large chunks of modern human endeavour and establishment. They form the important building blocks of our society. Without effective regulators, chaos is inevitable. Sad but true, India is proving to be no exception.

Health care takes up a major proportion of human time and effort and as an industry, it is probably even more complex than the global financial industry. It comprises a huge number of players across countries, all interlinked through a web of professionals and rich and powerful multinational drug corporates, hundreds of thousands of clinics, nursing homes and hospitals, medical colleges and universities, networks of academicians and academic bodies, governments, independent regulators, the World Health Organization, and the public at large. No surprise then that effective health care has so far proved an elusive concept in India.

Issues faced by individual doctors and patients are often intrinsic sometimes global. You could take a superficial view of things, whereby the ensuing blame game would further damage the profession. Alternatively, you could take a view that human behaviour across civilizations and nations on the planet follows similar patterns and if some countries can develop an effective and accountable health care system, India can too.

The Medical Council of India

With the powers vested in it by the law, the Medical Council of India (MCI) is the official regulator of doctors and medical education in our country. It is the job of this body to ensure that any doctor you consult meets a minimum standard of education and training. It has the powers to ensure that doctors follow its ethical code of conduct and those who go astray are disciplined. It has a legal responsibility to protect the interests of the patients.

It is an extremely important institution for India and Indians. If we believe that a large number of our doctors are either incompetent or unethical, the MCI is to be held responsible for such a scenario.

Not long ago, the MCI faced serious allegations of corruption, and that you could say is the universal fate of all government-owned or government-controlled institutions in this country. Inadequate resources, lack of transparency, very little monitoring or accountability, absence of an effective complaint system, and a politician- or power-centric approach rather than a public-centric approach can only indicate one thing—that our government establishment, nearly seventy years after Independence, is still working only for itself and not for the people of India. Prior to 1947, foreign rulers may have systematically encouraged this attitude but today, all citizens of our land must accept the blame for allowing the status quo to continue for this long.

It is not corruption (which now runs so rampant in our establishment that we have accepted it as routine part of our life) but incompetence that is a bigger problem in India. Our acceptance of the sub-standard is so deep-rooted that we have an even higher tolerance for it than for corruption. Incompetence has reached such epidemic proportions that bureaucrats and government officials often find it easier to do nothing at all, which is the most effective way of minimizing mistakes.

1. The Medical Register

One of the most important duties of a medical regulator is to maintain an accurate, transparent, conveniently searchable medical register. Anyone should be able to find out easily whether a person claiming to be a doctor is actually registered as a doctor and whether or not he is fit to practise medicine. A patient has the full right to know whether a doctor is being investigated or has been disciplined in the past, whether the specialist he is about to see is a genuine certified specialist. The people of India rely upon the MCI to do this job properly and make such information easily obtainable. But the current medical register maintained by the MCI is not fit for purpose. I will say no more.

I am not talking about sending a satellite into space (and that, by the way, we Indians are doing reasonably well, which just goes to show what can be accomplished under the right leadership); I am simply talking about developing and maintaining an effective database on the worldwide web. I could go into the boring details as to how the current one is incomplete, inaccurate, unhelpful, impossible to use, and so on, but that would only be worth doing if the powers that be were open to taking feedback.

2. Medical Education and Training

It is the responsibility of the MCI to ensure the upkeep and raising of standards in medical education and training in India, to monitor that medical colleges give out degrees that are fit for purpose and that every doctor in the country meets a minimum benchmark.

It has to ensure that the facilities it approves for medical teaching meet the set standards, have an appropriate faculty-student ratio, and are backed up by a well-equipped hospital with 'real' patients.

The MCI must keep a check that qualifications are being issued only to those who are adequately skilled to practise as doctors. I find it pathetic when it is said that the standard of medical education can be excused simply because we have hundreds of thousands of quacks in a country as vast as ours. Sooner or later, we will have to accept that small problems should not be ignored just because there are bigger ones out there. For it is these small problems that will grow into big ones tomorrow. I have argued elsewhere for a national level entry and exit examination to set a basic standard of medical education in the country.

Admittedly, our undergraduate medical education scenario could be better and there are some students who become doctors but certainly don't deserve to treat patients. In my opinion, our undergraduate system does work and produces doctors who are employable and are employed all over the world. It is the postgraduate education and training space that we particularly need to devote our attention to. It is in complete disarray and indicative, I think, of the momentous failure on the part of the MCI. There are absolutely no mechanisms in place to guarantee every doctor an opportunity for postgraduate training before being allowed to practise independently. Even those who do find limited places for specialty training are being let down. The duration of specialty training is too short, compared to the global average, and there are no guarantees that colleges and institutions are churning out qualified doctors who deserve to be called 'specialists'.

In other countries, specialty training takes around five-ten years, compared to two-three years in India. I can understand when professors in medical colleges say they are given too short a time to train and transform medical students into real specialists; it is impractical and impossible to achieve. For example, as a general surgeon myself, I know for a fact that you can't have a specialist ready for work in three years. Yet, this is what actually happened. I was given a specialty degree with licence to perform a wide array of surgeries on real human beings after a three-year training period. I can honestly tell you that when I received that degree, I was not fit to practise surgery as an independent surgeon. And I didn't. I obtained further training in different countries for another ten years before taking up my current consultant job within the National Health Service of UK. You could argue this was too long and that it should be possible to produce a general surgeon quicker than that. Still, I do think three years is too less a time period and many surgeons I have spoken to in Indian government institutions feel that the duration should be made six years with a mandatory three-year senior residency for people aiming to become general surgeons. There is no reason why the M.S. qualification cannot be issued as it is being done currently, but the licence to practise surgery as an independent specialist must only be conferred on completion of a further three years of structured training and demonstrated competence in performance of a number of procedures typically expected of a surgeon. Reforms are required and the MCI must lead the way, or who else will?

In other countries, training programmes are required to justify taking on trainees; it is not their birth right to have young professionals at their disposal as slaves, which seems to be the mind-set of faculty in many government institutions in India. In the UK and the US, only those places that are fit to impart training are accorded with the privilege and the honour of having a trainee; others just have to manage without them. Naturally then, programmes compete with each other in a healthy manner to make sure they provide a worthwhile training experience for trainees.

In India, trainees have no choice and no voice. They are completely at the mercy of professors, whether or not they are being trained properly. Just as the patient's voice is missing in our health care scene, the trainee's voice is largely missing in our education system. I am not saying students should tell teachers what to do. I am just saying students should be able to voice their grievances, and only those faculty in government medical colleges who have genuine interest in training the future generation have the privilege and the honour of doing so. GMC in the UK often conducts trainee surveys to gauge the mood of students and trainees across the country. These surveys often prove to be the drivers for change. In India, there are no such mechanisms and if you refuse to help your professor with his imminent Medical Association elections or his private case, you do so at your own peril. The examination system that awards postgraduate degrees is such that you may not obtain any qualification without the support of the college faculty. And the external examiners, whose job it is to ensure that the exams conducted are fair and robust, are usually only too happy with the honour of being an external examiner; if they disagree with the local faculty, they may not be invited to examine again.

A Hospital (Clinical Establishment) Regulator

Even though the MCI does not do much, at least we have somebody to regulate doctors. What about hospitals, who regulates them? What mechanisms do we have to monitor the working standards of hospitals? How do we know that a hospital has the required infrastructure and the desired number of doctors and nurses? How do we keep a check that hospitals don't advertise unethically? How do we ensure hospitals compete with each other in a healthy manner and not profiteer at the expense of poor patients?

It is common knowledge that we simply do not have any way of monitoring hospitals in India. It's not just the private sector hospitals I am talking about. Many public sector hospitals treat patients in establishments that are like slums among the hospital community and don't even deserve to be called hospitals.

There is dire need for hospitals and nursing homes to be regulated too. The private sector has offered alternatives where the government has failed. The National Accreditation Board for Hospital and Health care Providers (NABH) is one such Indian organization. Among international ones, accreditation by the Joint Commission International (JCI) is being used widely in the industry as a benchmark of satisfactory standards. These benchmarks have hence evolved to serve the shared needs of hospitals and patients. These private organizations have elaborate structures and I am confident they are driving up overall standards. However, they have no means of punishing the hospitals other than to deny them their seal of approval. They have no real power or authority. After all, there is a limit to what non-governmental organizations can do. The private sector can at best complement government efforts; it cannot replace it. There is no alternative to good governance and established regulatory systems. India is a perfect case in point.

It is worth mentioning here that the government of India has also realized the need for a regulator that will keep an eye on clinical facilities. The Clinical Establishments (Registration and Regulation) Act of 2010 is the first step in this direction. For the purposes of this Act, a clinical establishment is defined as 'a hospital, maternity home, nursing home, dispensary, clinic, sanatorium, or any other institution that offers services, facilities requiring diagnosis, treatment or care for illness, injury, deformity, abnormality or pregnancy in any recognized system of medicine. It also includes laboratory and diagnostic centre or any other place where pathological, bacteriological, genetic, radiological, chemical, biological investigations or other services with aid of laboratory or other medical equipment are carried out.'

Interestingly, it covers all kinds of clinical establishments, irrespective of which system of medicine they deal in and who owns them (including even the government and charitable facilities). But because health is a state subject according to the Constitution of India, it is not binding on the states. States can choose to adopt it by passing a resolution in their legislative assembly. As of September 2015, only nine states (Arunachal Pradesh, Himachal Pradesh, Mizoram, Sikkim, Uttar Pradesh, Bihar, Rajasthan, Jharkhand and Uttarakhand) and the Union Territories have adopted the Act. The Act makes provisions for a national and a state council which will maintain a register of all premises, define basic minimum standards, and develop a mechanism for collection and reporting of some statistics. One can see how with the important safeguards in constitution of councils, autonomy, accountability and appropriate (and largely independent) funding, this act could prove to be a game changer. Let us not raise our hopes too high, for given the current provisions, it will certainly not deliver on any of its objectives.

Current plans for constitution of its twenty-member national council, led by officers of Government of India and various other elected bodies, do not inspire confidence that this regulatory body will be any different from the existing ones. Moreover, by bringing in establishments involving AYUSH medicine in its fold, the government is further legitimizing quackery and degrading the standards of medicine in this country. No matter what the Indian government feels, in its current state, AYUSH establishments don't deserve to be treated on par with our hospitals. We have to decide if we are going to be a modern, scientific society that goes with established evidence or a society of sages that will cling on to the past.

As I have said before, modern medicine is an all-inclusive system that contains within it every single treatment that can testify to the rigours of science. All else is just tradition and belief, something that I cannot personally endorse in any form. Though currently this is not clearly stated, it is not obvious if councils will be aided by large teams that will carry out regular inspections of facilities to be able to deliver on the provisions of the Act. Moreover, it is not clear if there will be any additional funding provision in addition to what will be generated via fees charged from the establishment for registration. Needless to say, huge amounts of resources will be required for a regulator that must oversee all clinical establishments in a country as large as India. Without an autonomous council, adequate resources, accountability to the public and patients, regular as well as surprise inspections, and the desire as well as authority to implement punitive measures when necessary, it will degenerate into yet another corrupt, red tape-bound organization in the country.

Regulation of the Pharmaceutical and Medical Devices Industry

The pharmaceutical industry adds huge value to society and most benefits of modern medicine boil down to the periodic discovery of new drugs and devices. Without these, it would be impossible to practise medicine as we know it today. At the same time, the drug industry is a conglomerate of profit-seeking corporates whose primary interest is to improve their bottom line. Whether or not a majority of customers can afford their drugs does not concern them as long as the drugs bring them substantial profits. They openly admit that they make drugs for the developed world; so if people in countries like India, where these drugs are increasingly being tested prior to launch, cannot afford them, the industry could not care less.

The pharmaceutical industry cannot be trusted with people's health, as corporate greed has no limit. But many Western countries have developed systematic mechanisms to benefit from it rather than curb it. If the benefit comes at the cost of the poor in other parts of the world, it is not really a problem for them. Switzerland has developed mechanisms for banking of black money from all over the world. The Swiss benefit from offering a safe haven for corrupt money pouring in from all over the world. These are the same governments that are often heard preaching the highest moral codes to the rest of the world. I for one don't for a moment believe Indians need any lessons in morality.

It is true that most of the continuing medical education programmes and conferences in India (and probably in the rest of the world) are organized with industry support. It may also be true that a large number of doctors in India first hear about a new drug from the company representative and not a scientific journal. After all, reading scientific articles is not actually cheap when you live and work in a developing country. A typical article can cost anywhere between USD 25–50 and hundreds of thousands of articles are published every year. Take it from me, you need to read more than one article to keep abreast of the latest developments.

I have argued elsewhere in this book how India needs to develop its own open access publishing platforms, where Indian researchers can freely share ideas, thoughts and research. (My competing interests, as a co-founder of WebmedCentral, a publishing platform, need to be noted here). Much like other industries, the publishing and research industry is also systematically controlled by Western institutions and unsurprisingly, they use this power to pursue their own agenda and ambition. They decide what research is acceptable, which journals are important and who can publish in them. This in turn decides which institutions and academics are important. These numbers then perpetuate a cycle where Indian institutions cannot even dream of achieving a level playing field with their Western counterparts, academically speaking, which in turn means they lose out in terms of attracting meritorious students and hundreds of billions of dollars of research money. The world of scientific research and academia is like a closed club and developing countries like India are simply not allowed entry. I have suggested creating a separate club where Indian researchers are not hostage to Western journals for visibility and developing Indian benchmarks of ranking academics that look beyond the flawed world of 'impact factors'.

There is a bigger question to answer here. We have to decide as a society if we really want to outsource the business of continuing medical education to the drug industry. For if we do, we can be sure that companies will only sponsor events that promote their own products. Researchers will continue to be sponsored depending on which companies' products they endorse. Conferences will continue to be supported depending on the relationship between conference organizers and corporates. Leaving education to corporates will mean that they will use it as a platform to showcase their products in the best possible light. For example, when a company representative tells you about their new innovative drug to fight a cancer, they may selectively quote evidence from the scientific literature that supports this drug; in the process, scientific balance is lost and facts misrepresented.

An alternative system could be engendered where doctors organize such events for each other as they currently do, but neither the organizers nor the doctors attending these conferences would get any sponsorship from the corporates. Doctors would hate it, and this is one reason even Western countries have not yet been able to implement something like this. But we in India can come up with our own rules to protect our people. It may mean that doctors will be able to attend and organize fewer conferences. The cynic in me feels that it might not be a bad thing. Having said that, I have no problem with doctors attending and hosting such events as long as they can bear the costs themselves without any help from corporates.

When a company knows it can sell more goods by bribing or incentivizing doctors in one of the many recognized ways (sponsorship to organize meetings or conferences, sponsorship to attend meetings, industry sponsored fellowships, etc.), it will do so. Obviously, the industry as a whole loses out and so does society, but that cannot concern an individual medical representative whose job depends on selling a particular medicine. That is why markets need regulators, otherwise everyone loses. It is a fact that distorted markets not only harm the consumers but also the competing players.

If we had an effective regulator for drug companies, it would be able to prevent them from bribing doctors and punish them robustly when caught doing so. With an effective regulator, drug companies would not be able to treat unsuspecting poor Indians like guinea pigs when they conduct trials. We could force them to follow Western standards of safety and give out reasonable compensations when accidents happen. An effective regulator would ensure quality control for all the drugs and devices manufactured in India. Now, I am not sure whether you are aware that we do have a regulator for the pharmaceutical industry in India. It is the Central Drugs Standard Control Organization (CDSCO). But it is so severely under-resourced and understaffed that it cannot even control the counterfeit drug industry, let alone enforce an ethical code of conduct that, frankly, even many Western countries are struggling to implement.

Given the fact that India's successful generic drug industry is now the world's only reliable source for inexpensive life-saving drugs, it is not just in the interest of Indian people but all the poor across the world that we effectively monitor and regulate our pharmaceutical industry. They are doing a good job on the whole and they need our support. According to a recent report by Deloitte: 'India today has 546 facilities approved by the Food and Drug Administration of USA (USFDA), 857 facilities approved by the Medicines and Health Care Regulatory Authority of UK (UKMHRA), and 1,259 facilities approved by WHO-GMP.' Though companies regulated by Western countries naturally aim at maintaining high standards, thousands of local companies catering only to the domestic market are operating at will in a market where there is no effective regulator. This has meant that doctors are not sure of the quality of many medicines afloat in the market and are often forced to rely on more expensive brands.

This has also meant that the market is riddled with combination pills that have no rationale and result in overprescription and overuse of drugs. The Drug Controller General of India himself admitted that our regulatory framework needs to be strengthened while pointing out that by the end of 2013, the Indian regulator will have 327 employees compared to 14,000 employed by the USFDA.

The USFDA had a budget of US$ 4.5 billion for 2015, 2.6 billion of which was contributed by the government while the rest was generated through user fees from the industry. Similarly, the UKMHRA employs over 1, 200 people and is funded partly by the government, with the rest coming from the pharmaceutical industry in the form of fees. It will generate an operational surplus of £20 million this year pitted against an income of £150 million. The majority of the income was generated via fees, with contribution from the government's department of health being £28.5 million. Western countries know how to keep their public institutions financially viable and more or less independent. India will sooner or later need to develop these mechanisms. A regulator can only be held accountable and hold others accountable when it has the resources to deliver on the promises made and is free from bureaucratic clutches.

India needs an effective drug regulator to maintain the reputation of its large generic drug industry, especially as the protectionist tendency of Western governments invariably means that instances of poor quality that come to light will be systematically blown out of proportion in the world media. We should use any such criticism to improve the standards of this industry and to support our drug makers in fighting the multinational corporate giants out there. The alternative is chaos, as even essential medicines would be out of reach for the ordinary Indian citizen. At the same time, the industry should be allowed to make reasonable profits where they have enough money to meet regulatory requirements, develop new drugs and generate profits for shareholders. Conflicting interests of different stakeholders need to be carefully balanced. An effective, accountable, transparent regulator can achieve this. A plethora of regulations, without the will to implement anything, and corrupt officials willing to turn a blind eye to everything will harm everybody—the patients, the industry, and of course, the reputation of our country as a manufacturing base.

There is some talk of a separate medical devices regulator in India and I wonder if it is entirely necessary. Both the FDA and the MHRA have regulation of medical devices within their remit. The medical devices industry is essential to modern medicine. Though, currently, a majority of the products are imported, there is no reason why that must remain so for a country with one-fifth of the world's population that aspires to be a global hub for medical care. With the right environment and suitable incentives, the industry can make these devices in India.

Many single-use devices are used on multiple patients, disregarding safety precautions. Individual surgeons are powerless as systems have evolved where single-use devices have to be used again and again to keep the treatments affordable for Indian patients. Individuals can only be as honest as the rest of the society will allow them to be. Try to be more honest than the rest, and you will be labelled an impractical idealist. And if you're any less honest than expected of you, you are sure to be labelled corrupt. Each of us has to toe the fine line between realism and idealism, as decided for us by others. Whilst we all believe that we ourselves completely govern our actions, the truth is that the actions of individuals are usually determined by the principles and ethos of the society they live in. Societies in turn change very slowly, only when a critical number of people assemble the courage to challenge prevailing notions and widely held beliefs.

The National Pharmaceutical Pricing Authority (NPPA) controls prices of pharmaceutical products in our country. In many ways, it is doing a more effective job than many Western regulators, in terms of protecting the interests of the vulnerable sections of society. But it is also required to ensure that the industry continues to be profitable and attractive. If the Indian pharmaceutical sector does not have the resources to invest in monitoring and safety mechanisms, the NPPA will have to share part of the burden. It is a tricky balance to achieve and regulators can easily make a mistake on either side. So it is important that external bodies and agencies not only give feedback to the regulator but also monitor it. For this, the regulator needs to be open and transparent in its functioning.

I am all for the protection of intellectual property as long as intellectuals recognize the contribution of global societies. For example, it is unfair to deny benefits of academic exercise to the vast population of India when Western countries systematically benefit from the work of millions of Indians educated at the expense of the Indian taxpayer. Intellectuals also need to recognize that they benefit from the collective pool of human knowledge accumulated over many millennia, long before these patents and rights were invoked. Fairness in the modern world order has many facets of discussion and any comprehensive discussion of intellectual property rights needs to take a holistic view of the situation.

The Pharmacy Regulator

The Pharmacy Council of India (PCI), much like the MCI, is a statutory body under the Government of India, constructed under the Pharmacy Act of 1948. The council is constituted by the Central government with elected, nominated and ex-officio members.

The main function of the PCI is to determine standards of education and maintain a register of pharmacists. It is its job to ensure institutions imparting education in pharmacy are fit for this purpose.

There is another regulator involved here—the All India Council for Technical Education (AICTE)—which was made a statutory body as per the AICTE Act of 1987. This body too is involved in regulation of pharmacy education and, according to some, this has further compounded the situation with the net result of two responsible regulators in operation where neither works effectively.

Now, this book is not about pharmacists and I know little about the profession, but the problems are largely similar. With nearly 90 per cent of pharmacists now trained in private institutions, standards are slipping. Mechanisms to ensure that all graduating pharmacists possess adequate knowledge, have opportunities for continued education, and that people other than trained pharmacists cannot dispense (sell is a more appropriate word in the Indian context) medicines do not exist.

Just as any human being who wants to call himself a doctor is free to do so in India (this is what freedom of expression and democracy has sadly come to mean in this country), any human being who can match a doctor's handwriting on a prescription note with the name of the medicine on a box can dispense medicines.

Licences to obtain retail and wholesale chemist shops are issued by the CDSCO and though the licences are probably issued to a qualified person, we all know that most medicines in India are dispensed like groceries by low paid workers with no real knowledge of pharmacy. We also know that anybody can go and buy any medicine from any chemist shop in the country, even without a prescription. In such a situation, it will sound impractical if I even talk about preventing quacks from prescribing modern medicine as at least then the pharmacy can fall back on the valid excuse that they cannot distinguish between doctors and quacks.

In Western countries, pharmacists make sure that drugs prescribed by doctors don't mix with each other or with something else that the patient is on. It also falls to the pharmacists to ensure that patients understand how and when the medicines should be consumed. But in a country where everybody is allowed to dispense medicines, the real pharmacists have neither role nor responsibility. A pharmacy degree is only important because it is a necessary formality to be fulfilled in order to set up a chemist shop. Apart from that, it is hard to differentiate a pharmacy from a general store and indeed, in many places in the country, the two comfortably coexist.

Though reforms concerning systems governing the quality of education and the standard of regulators will be fundamental to any attempt at remedying the situation, some concrete steps could be taken tomorrow. All the CDSCO needs to do is to conduct 100 surprise checks and de-licence premises where medicines are being dispensed by anybody other than a pharmacist or if scheduled drugs are being dispensed without the prescription of a doctor with his registration number on it. Our regulatory bodies don't believe active screening of abuse of the system is their job, and this attitude needs to change if India wishes to see a positive change in regulatory culture. The prevalent culture where our regulatory bodies happily bury their heads in the sand and only ever react passively to complaints is at the root of a number of failures in our democratic society. Reforms in the profession of pharmacy have to go hand in hand with reforms in the medical profession for any real impact to be visible.

The Nursing Regulator

Similar to regulators overseeing other health care professionals, the Indian Nursing Council (INC) is an 'autonomous' body set up under the Indian Nursing Council Act of 1947 to establish a uniform standard of training for nurses, midwives and health visitors. Let me give you an idea of the current state of affairs. Out of the 1,491 nursing schools registered with the council for the ANM (Auxiliary Nursing Midwifery Diploma) course alone, only 142 are government institutions. The rest are distributed between charitable and private sectors. Then there are the GNM (General Nursing and Midwifery), B.Sc, M.Sc, and M. Phil courses. We all know that the performance quality of nurses in India, much like that of doctors and pharmacists, is hugely variable, with standards being pathetically low in many places and world class in others.

Pretty much every hospital that has struggled to meet its requirement of nurses has opened its own nursing school. As India needs millions of nurses, this would be all right as long as we could ensure that the entry and exit criteria were robust. In absence of such benchmarks, we are simply penalizing well-trained, dedicated, talented nurses by making them compete with anybody who knows how to wear the uniform. The problem is further compounded by a number of qualifications with no clear demarcation of jurisdiction. How can you have clear jurisdiction in a country for different types of nurses where hundreds of thousands of quacks regularly infringe on the jurisdiction of doctors? The end result is massive migration of good nurses out of India to countries that value their qualification, give them the respect they deserve, and provide respectable remuneration.

We must not allow our educational qualifications to be so diluted that there is little incentive to obtaining them, and that is a fundamental aspect to examine not just in the education of doctors, nurses and pharmacists in India but in every single walk of life. As a result of dilution of standards, the nursing profession in India has been reduced to the standard of domestic workers in many places. In some places, you could argue domestic workers are paid more and treated better than nurses. Now, I do believe our domestic workers need to be treated on par with others in society, but I was hoping we would achieve that by improving their lot and not diminishing that of others.

Constitution of a Regulator

A truly effective regulator needs some legal authority backing it. This is not a problem in India as our regulators, when they exist, carry the authority of a parliamentary act. What a regulator also needs is representation from all sections of society whilst maintaining subject matter knowledge and freedom from undue government influence. In India, such freedom is especially important as sooner or later, every state organization becomes corrupt. Even the so-called autonomous institutions in India are not free from bureaucratic clutches and that is one big reason educational and other institutions in India are held back.

It would seem obvious that any organization claiming to regulate and control doctors has at least an equal representation from lay public, just as the GMC of UK (six out of its twelve council members are lay people) does. This does not apply to India though. The MCI has many more members than its counterparts elsewhere in the world and almost all of them are doctors. Out of ninety-four council members and ten executive committee members that I counted on their website on 22 August 2015, I could not find even one who was not a doctor. Naturally, doctors look out for each other and offending doctors are never booked. The rare occasions when they are, punishment is not really proportionate and hardly a deterrent.

Most council members are elected by people in the medical profession itself and this clearly lies at the root of the problem. Would doctors elect you to discipline them? If you treated doctors harshly, would you be re-elected? This is in sharp contrast to the GMC of UK whose members are appointed by an external body.

A regulator can only be truly independent if people overseeing its daily activities are appointed on the basis of their talent and interest in the field, and if its executive members come from a cross section of interested parties, including the public. Finally, they must be held responsible for failures. There is no doubt that some council members will represent the profession that the regulator intends to regulate, but forming councils comprising entirely of the regulated will fail for obvious reasons. The MCI is a perfect example.

Funding of a Regulator

The General Medical Council of United Kingdom does not get any state funding and is funded almost entirely through annual registration fees paid by the doctors. In lieu, it provides efficient service to both doctors and patients. Just looking at the website of the Medical Council of India, on the other hand, will give you an idea of the quality of service they provide. The MCI has no system of charging annual fees from doctors. Indeed, it does not even know where doctors are located and whether they are dead or alive! It is largely funded by the money it takes from private medical colleges for granting them registration.

Though regulators across the world operating in different fields are part funded by the governments, one can see how this eventually (perhaps more so in India than in other countries) translates into political control and loss of autonomy. A truly independent regulator must be able to generate its own finances, and this can usually only come from charging those it regulates. We in India need to think about how we wish to fund our regulators. The government could provide a one-time upfront establishment cost and subsequent public sector contributions could be kept at a minimum, even zero. Whichever mechanism we go for, the crucial factors are going to be autonomy and accountability. The regulators must be made to account for every paisa they generate and spend. Without these functional mechanisms to regulate the regulator, the system is likely to collapse, as it has in India.

The Way Forward

The health care mess in India is a failure of policy.
—Dr Gita Sen, IIM Bangalore

India needs to reorganize its health care system.
—World Health Organization

It is never going to be easy to provide adequate health care to 1.2 billion people, and anyone who pretends otherwise either does not understand India or how health care works. The task is so enormous that just the thought of it can be immobilizing. All I have tried to do in this book is to give you a snapshot of the health care system in India and the challenges it faces. It is possible that your impression of reality is not as unsettling as my portrayal of it. It is also possible you don't agree with everything I say. But none of us can deny the need for improvement, and that is the ultimate objective of this book. The task I set out to do would remain incomplete if I didn't even attempt to suggest steps to rectify the situation, to create hope for a better tomorrow.

Before enumerating what should be done, it is worth acknowledging that these suggestions are interdependent. So implementing them selectively may prove counterproductive. If you have somehow landed straight onto this chapter and find it slightly abrupt, that might be because I have made a case for these reforms in other sections of this book.

1. **Radically Reform the Medical Council of India:** Currently, the MCI is ineffective in every single domain of responsibility it shoulders. It needs radical transformation. So much so that I think we should dismantle the current body and create a new, autonomous MCI with a considerably smaller council. The council should have equal representation from doctors and others in society and its members should be appointed through a robust selection process overseen by another independent panel (similar to the GMC of UK), rather than elected from amongst the existing pool of doctors (as is currently the case). The MCI also needs to be fortified with resources in order to be able to carry out its responsibilities. There is no reason why it could not be partly or completely funded through annual fees paid by doctors. A reformed MCI will need to urgently work on the areas outlined below.

   a. **Medical Register:** Creating a fit-for-purpose medical register that is accurate and easily searchable. It should provide details about every qualified doctor, their fitness to practise, details of any ongoing or concluded disciplinary proceedings, area of specialization, place of work, etc.
   b. **Renewed Practical Code:** As we saw in Chapter 1, the MCI needs to come up with a new practical code that correctly represents the realities of the twenty-first century. Only then will it be able to implement it and regulate the profession effectively.

c. **Robustly Tackle Departures from Code:** The MCI needs to develop mechanisms to work with a team of inspectors in every state who actively look out for doctors engaging in unethical and fraudulent behaviour. Such people should then be thoroughly investigated and handed robust, deterring punishments. In some cases, a ban for prolonged periods or even for life may be appropriate.

d. **Develop a Culture of Self-audit amongst Doctors:** Clinical governance and auditing of doctors' results are unheard of in India. The MCI needs to encourage a culture where every doctor must study at least one aspect of his/her clinical practice every year and publish the data. As per my suggestions of free publishing all medical data in a climate of post-publication peer review, publishing such data could be done at the click of a button in a very transparent and cost-effective way.

e. **National Entrance Test for Admission to All Government and Private Medical Colleges:** As discussed earlier, I think the idea of a national entrance test, the NEET, is good and worth implementing in a careful manner with sufficient warning to states and students. The scores of such a test could then be used by individual medical colleges for determining their intake. It will eventually mean that students will not have to sit a number of long examinations. Nevertheless, if any individual college or state wishes to supplement the information from national scores with a further brief test or interview of its own, it must be allowed to do so.

Private medical colleges should broadly be able to decide for themselves whom they offer places to, but it is reasonable to ask them to allocate a fair proportion (approximately 25 per cent) of their seats towards government quotas. Moreover, there is no reason why government medical colleges should not have freedom to offer some of their seats to Non Resident Indians (NRIs) or international students for a higher fee. Naturally, the proportion will be much lower, perhaps up to 25 per cent.

f. **Give Medical Colleges Independence in Determining Fees:** Whilst insisting they maintain their charitable status, private medical colleges should be allowed to decide what fees they charge students. Underfunded institutions cannot impart top quality education and would find themselves unable to compete globally. It would only be fair that students from India and those from a poorer background pay lower fees than do international students and NRIs. Additionally, there should also be a large number of means-tested bursaries and development of student loans. These measures could then gradually be rolled out in government-run medical colleges as well, to prevent them from becoming second-class institutions in terms of quality and infrastructure. By and large, we need to give our medical colleges (both private and government-owned) much more independence in deciding their fees and student intake, training our focus instead on implementing norms related to structure, standard of education and patient care. They should also have freedom to recruit faculty from around the world and to pay them whatever the market rates demand.

g. **Creating a National Exit Test:** A national exit test binding on all medical colleges will set a uniform minimum acceptable standard that all new entrants to the profession must achieve. Because the level of education obtainable in medical colleges (both public and private) can be extremely variable, we need a national exit test before students can be called doctors. This will put pressure on institutions to ensure their students are fit to actually practise medicine once they graduate. Such an assessment of the quality of medical education obtained through an exit test would need to go beyond a simple MCQ format. There is no reason why the scores of such an exit test could not also be used to allocate places for further postgraduate training, which I believe must be mandatory before students can practise independently. Naturally, it can only be implemented if we can guarantee further training to all the medical students. Numbers for each postgraduate area of training could be determined depending on what the population needs. For example, it is conceivable that more than half will of the students will head for training in General Practice.

h. **Separate Committee with Postgraduate Training Focus Groups for Each Medical Specialty including General Practice:** Creating such Focus Groups will determine duration and format of postgraduate training for each medical specialty and will be responsible for certifying that specialists are fit for purpose. It will also ensure that we train the number of specialists that we actually need in this country.

   Furthermore, this committee should work with private hospitals, nursing homes and clinics to create a wide-ranging web of adequately remunerated, postgraduate training jobs where we can offer opportunities for further training to each and every medical graduate in the country. It is not impossible for us to create a system similar to the National Resident Matching Programs in USA. Such a programme could use the score of the national exit examination to rank students. Again, it is possible that various institutions may wish to have some control over who enters their premises.

Finally, the continuing medical education of doctors in their specialty (another area that is in a mess today) should be left to these Specialty Focus Groups who can work out a suitable arrangement to take care of this process. These Specialty Focus Groups can play a hugely important role in regulating such training and continued education.

i. **Open a Patient Complaint Cell:** The voice of the patient is completely missing in Indian health care. You have no recourse against a doctor if things go wrong. You can take the legal route but you probably know how efficient our legal machinery is. In other countries, you can complain against an individual doctor or hospital to the respective regulator, but not in India. Here, you can do nothing. Without empowering the patient, there is nobody to question a doctor or a hospital when errors occur and they operate with complete impunity and no accountability.

It is not too difficult for the MCI to open a patient cell where patients can freely complain against doctors. Official awareness about problems may even force the MCI to investigate and take action. I am not saying every doctor will need to be disciplined for every complaint but having a robust mechanism that gives the patient the option of lodging a formal complaint could instil fear in the minds of unethical doctors who, at the moment, are able to get away with anything.

Only when we do have such established mechanisms in place to regulate the profession, will it be appropriate to take medicine out of consumer courts. Medicine is not a business and patients are not consumers. Encouraging such a culture benefits nobody and only leads to overuse of diagnostic tests and practice of defensive medicine. The end result would be expensive health care, which we should all be keen to avoid. Otherwise, we could have a scenario like that in USA, where the country spends nearly 2.5 times the money on health care (public and private expenditure combined) that many European countries do, and still finds itself unable to provide reasonable health care for all. The UK government spends as much as USA does on health care, in terms of public spending as a proportion of the GDP, and provides health care free for all at the point of delivery. USA can never dream of doing this because fear of litigation and excessive greed has made health care extremely expensive.

2. **Establish Indian Institute for Clinical Excellence:** Science is incontrovertible but, often, scientific evidence is not. Scientists increasingly use the tools of mathematics and statistics, but they understand little to prove their hunches and hypotheses; it is now a fact that many a time, published scientific findings and results are plain wrong. And all doctors know it, or they should know it. We never base our clinical decisions on one study. We need to see results replicated by different researchers across the population before they are incorporated into routine clinical practice. We also know that there may be negative results never published, so we speak

to colleagues and also look at our own experiences. Sooner or later, the lie gets caught and the truth survives. Moreover, a good doctor then weighs the condition of the individual patient, his social circumstances, finances and personal situation in life so as to give appropriate advice. Medical decision-making is a complex algorithmic process and yet, it is more than just an algorithm. It must also imbibe compassion, kindness and a sense of duty.

However, it is also true that doctors can rarely think beyond their patients and themselves. Each one of us will happily spend the entire health care budget on the patients we look after. Ask a bone marrow transplant specialist and he will tell you no amount of money is too much to save a child dying of leukaemia. We are all passionate people, and that in itself isn't a bad thing. Society, though, cannot make important decisions on the basis of emotion. It needs to balance a number of conflicting priorities and come up with ways and means whereby individual goals and aspirations can be transformed into attainable objectives for the group as a whole.

This is why doctors need guidelines in routine areas of complex medical practice. In the UK, NICE (National Institute for Health and Care Excellence) does this job. It forms advisory groups whose job is to come up with recommendations that professionals and managers can then use for patient care and planning. NICE decides which treatments apply to the British population and what is cost effective for the British health care system as a whole. Overall, NICE has a huge responsibility to match the efforts of the medical profession, the industry and the government with the needs of the patients. These advisory guidelines often include research ideas. If the advisory group feels that the evidence in a certain area is too weak to enable a clear recommendation, they suggest more research is carried out before reaching a conclusion.

To meet these objectives, NICE has representation from professionals across a range of specialties, patients and lay groups. Guidelines constructed by NICE are valued not just within the UK but throughout the world. However, we must note that NICE makes these guidelines for British people. The institute takes into account what is a reasonable sum to spend to preserve a year of life for a patient in Britain, a very rich country compared to India. (NICE uses a threshold of GBP 20,000 for every Quality Adjusted Life Year saved for approving treatments and drugs.) People on the panel are British professionals, British people and British patients. India cannot and must not use NICE guidelines for the Indian population.

3. **Effective Clinical Establishments Regulator:** The Indian government needs to set up a separate regulator for all clinical establishments (hospitals, nursing homes, clinics and diagnostic laboratories) in the country. Current plans for the Clinical Establishments Regulator, as we saw in the last chapter, don't go far enough and have limited market penetration as such.

    a. **Autonomy and Funding:** The regulator will need to be autonomous and independent. It will also need to be adequately funded. It should not be too difficult to generate the required resources by charging establishments an annual fee.

b. **Updated Record of Facilities and Issue of Licences:** This regulator will maintain a clear record of the number of facilities, hospital beds, laboratories, clinics, etc. in each area and only issue licences for establishment of new clinics, laboratories and hospital beds in areas that need them. This will avoid oversupply in some areas and gross undersupply in others.

c. **Patient Complaint Cell:** This regulator will also maintain a Patient Complaint Cell where patients can complain against hospitals, diagnostic laboratories, clinics and nursing homes. All complaints will be appropriately investigated and deterrent punishments will be meted out to erring institutions.

d. **Accountability:** Such a regulator will also need to instill some sort of clinical accountability in the facilities it oversees. Asking them to submit data on mortality, average duration of hospital stay for different conditions, complication rates etc. will go a long way in improving the standards of clinical care in the country as will surprise checks and periodic case reviews.

e. **Infrastructure, Manpower and Licences:** It will need to enforce that hospitals and nursing homes have the required infrastructure and manpower. It will need to check that people are only licensed for the work they are fit to do and that licence statuses are periodically monitored.

f. **Fees and Revenue:** The regulator will determine appropriate consultation and procedure charge ranges to improve transparency and allow fair competition. We need a sustainable health care system where doctors, laboratories, nursing homes and hospitals can earn a reasonable amount of revenue. Nobody should be allowed to charge less or more than a certain amount. It goes without saying that any range will need to be fairly broad to allow for variations, but such a step seeks to acknowledge two broad facts—on one hand, profiteering and greed has no upper limit and on the other, and perhaps more importantly, underpaying professionals only encourages unethical behaviour.

4. **Role of the Government:** Health care is, by and large, a state responsibility and in almost all countries of the world, governments have embraced it. Without significant investment of time and money by the government, it would be impossible to even think of improving public health.

    a. **Increase Public Health Care Expenditure:** The first thing the government needs to do if it is really serious about the health of Indian public is to considerably increase expenditure on health care. Without doing this, the poor in the country cannot even dream of having access to anything that will remotely resemble modern health care. We may have to take small incremental steps but it is certain we will need to spend close to at least 5–6 per cent of our GDP to bring about a real change.
    b. **Overhaul Primary Health Centres (PHCs):** Our PHCs need urgent overhaul and significant investment. Doctors and other professionals need to be paid much more to attract them to dead-end career jobs in villages where there are no decent schools for children and no means of family entertainment. Each PHC should

also have a manager who will make sure that all non-medical things and organizational aspects are taken care of. This will help doctors to focus on patient care and implementation of a range of government programmes. As we have established earlier, it will need something like twice the current total of our health budget to be spent on our PHCs alone to bring about some real changes in Indian primary health care.

c. **More High Quality Medical Colleges:** It will not be possible for the Government of India to provide adequate inpatient hospital care for everybody in the near future, but it does have a responsibility to ensure there are high quality medical colleges in every part of the country. We already have world-class institutions like AIIMS in New Delhi and PGIMER in Chandigarh that are working well. Though we recognize that much can be done to improve these premier institutions too, it is obvious that state medical colleges don't even come close to them. We should reasonably aspire to bring all our medical colleges up to the level of AIIMS, if not make them better.

Moreover, we need to considerably increase the number of such facilities. I don't think it is unreasonable to vision a number close to one medical college per parliamentary constituency to be able to produce the amount of medical manpower India needs and will continue to need in future. It might mean upgrading many district general hospitals to medical colleges, which will in turn need significant planning and investment. So, while on one hand, the government will be spending a significant amount of money on PHCs, on the other hand, an equally huge investment will be required in establishing and upgrading medical colleges and their associated hospitals.

Faculty in these institutions will need to be paid world-class salaries in lieu of the expectation that they nurture a world-class research environment. Our government jobs need to become lucrative enough for us to be able to use the threat of dismissal effectively. The present environment, where nobody wants the job in the first place, doesn't give us any bargaining position really when it comes to demanding output.

d. **Consumer-Centric Approach:** The prevalent colonial mind-set in India, where government machinery think they are working for somebody else, needs to change and government institutions need to become much more responsive to the needs of the public. Having an effective reception counter and a mechanism for complaints that promises confidentiality will go a long way as a first step.

e. **Revised Concept of Community Health Centres (CHCs):** With all the complexities that characterize modern medicine, I think the traditional concept of a CHC is becoming somewhat irrelevant. You can only practise cutting-edge medicine in full-fledged hospitals. The old idea of a CHC serving as some sort of a medium-level facility is outdated. Ideally, we need to turn all CHCs into hospitals but currently, we do not have enough money or manpower to do this, so we mustn't waste any time even thinking about it. I also feel that if we can develop our PHCs considerably, they should be able to deal with a lot of what currently gets referred to CHCs. This will also mean that people get maximum health care closer to home.

f. **Develop Indian Research:** A society will never develop if a significant number of people are not thinking critically and scientifically. Indian doctors need to develop a critical and evidence-based approach to health care. It needs a gradual transformation in thinking. This should happen alongside development of adequately funded research facilities. The government needs to recognize that research needs upfront investment, which can only come from two sources—government and charities. In India, there are very few research charities, so there is no other alternative.
g. **Not to Confuse Quacks with Doctors:** Yes, it is true that a lot of poor Indians are forced to turn to quacks for help but to legalize this and give it a seal of approval is not much worse than writing off poor lives. If the government can make modern health care accessible and affordable, quacks will die a natural death. For all practical purposes, AYUSH professionals practising modern medicine are quacks.
h. **Develop an All India Ambulance Service:** Elsewhere in this book we have discussed the stark absence of ambulance services in the country. It is only fitting that a twenty-first century India develops a first-rate ambulance service that can at least look after patients in case of emergency. Telephone operators managing this service will keep a record of the bed availability status in all public and private sector hospitals. This will mean government hospitals will need to allocate a proportion of their beds for emergency patients. Private hospitals will also have to do the same. On paper, as part of a deal for all the concessions they get from the government, private hospitals are asked to reserve

some beds for poor patients, but mechanisms for poor patients to use these beds are not easy to find and private hospitals stand accused of not facilitating them when requirement arises. As part of a mesh of emergency beds, private hospitals won't be able to deny the use of these beds earmarked for public patients.

i. **Allow Government Institutions Autonomy to Generate Finances:** Not only regulatory institutions but even our medical colleges, universities and hospitals are inadequately funded and hence cannot compete with global institutions. There are many ways these institutions can raise money for themselves and we should encourage this so that they are able to engage in healthy competition with their counterparts elsewhere in the world.

j. **Provide Incentives for Opening Clinical Establishments in Underserved Areas:** The government has to realize that rural India is not exactly a place doctors are desperate to work in and hospitals may struggle just to recover costs. So it will need to make available significant public incentives to encourage private players and corporates to open hospitals, diagnostic laboratories and clinics in our smaller towns and villages. The government must facilitate land and also bear some of the setting up costs with perhaps a provision that the expenditure can be recovered from future profits. These facilities may also need tax breaks and resources to develop schools and other basic amenities for the families of doctors and nurses.

k. **Autonomous Regulatory Institutions:** Regulatory institutions can only work effectively when they are free of government control. The governing councils of regulators should represent a cross-section of Indian society alongside those with subject knowledge. Moreover, regulators need a degree of financial independence and resources to be able to function effectively. In modern societies, regulators have a very important function to carry out and to be really effective, they need to be autonomous and adequately funded.

1. **Take Steps to Reduce Corruption:** We all know that whenever we talk about anything to do with the public sector in India, corruption is the big elephant in the room. To say that we need to reduce it is like saying we need to become a rich country is equal to stating an aspiration. We need to think of systematic mechanisms such as those adopted by other countries to make this aspiration a reality. Transparency, accountability, effective complaint mechanisms and robust disciplinary procedures are some of the many things that will go some way in tackling systematic corruption in India.

5. **Reform and Resource Central Drugs Standard Control Organization (CDSCO):** The CDSCO is our drug regulator but it does not have the resources to tackle and regulate the huge pharmaceutical and medical devices industry. Whether or not we bring out a separate medical devices regulator or develop it under the wings of the CDSCO, the end objective is for drugs and devices manufactured in the country to meet adequate quality standards. The NPPA needs to ensure prices are set appropriately and there must be mechanisms in the system to prevent abuse. Furthermore, there should be a way to make the MRP of medicines and devices reflect

the manufacturing costs incurred. We should ban corporate funding of medical conferences, and corporate gifts and sponsorships to doctors in all forms. This will go some way in improving the work ethic in the profession.

6. **Migrating Doctors:** I am a migrant doctor myself and I think forcing doctors to work in India without ensuring that they have adequately paid jobs in hospitals and PHCs that resemble medical facilities will only worsen the problem. Once we have world-class mechanisms in place, it would be reasonable for the nation to ask those doctors who still want to migrate to compensate the system. It could be a sum of money that doctors agree to pay within five years of leaving India. This would be easily recovered if tied to passport renewal or visas. Moreover, they should be asked to continue making a contribution to Indian health care in some form. There are many ways India can tap into the huge pool of expatriate Indian medicos and use them for education, training and knowledge sharing.

7. **Pharmacy Reforms:** We need to pull up our pharmacies to a level where they are not mere grocery stores. A number of reforms are required here. First of all, for all scheduled drugs, they should be required to document the registration number of doctors and that should be recorded in a central database. Pharmacies should document the registration number of the doctors prescribing a scheduled drug. This should be recorded in a central database. Such a database will put some fear of irrational prescribing in the minds of doctors. Implementing generic prescribing is more aspiration than reality at present,

as how will pharmacists then decide which brand to dispense to a patient. However, it may be piloted with government institutions with a central mechanism for procuring, which will also give the government the ability to negotiate a cheaper settlement.

8. **Private Hospital Reforms:** We have discussed above some of the steps that need to be taken to regulate all types of clinical establishments. But when it comes to private hospitals and nursing homes, we need some more measures. Firstly, it is my view that all advertising, including that engaged in by hospitals and laboratories, should be prohibited. This will ensure that freelance independent doctors are not at a disadvantage compared to their colleagues working for corporate hospitals.

   Secondly, I think private hospitals should be asked to pay salaries to doctors without any targets or commissions. Such a move will recognize that it is not the responsibility of doctors to bring business and if a hospital is struggling to attract patients, it might be because it is in an area where either there are too many hospitals already or patients cannot afford to pay their charges. Getting rid of commissions will further make sure that doctors do not directly profit from declaring more and more of us as diseased.

   We have already talked about how we need to develop a culture of self-audit and monitoring amongst doctors and hospitals. It might need some encouragement from the respective regulators to internalize and act upon these ideas. In addition, private hospitals should be expected to help with training of junior doctors, which will eventually only help them as, universally, private hospitals struggle to recruit junior-level doctors. Finally, as discussed earlier, I would expect private hospitals to earmark a few beds for use by Local Ambulance/Emergency Services Networks in lieu of favours that the health care industry enjoys at the expense of the public.

9. **Indian Research Database—an IndMed:** The world of science, research and academics is an industry working very closely with universities, corporates and governments. You control this world and you forever reap the benefits of all the academic developments mankind will see. Unsurprisingly, these are closely guarded fiefdoms that are difficult to break into.

   Scientists need to be able to publish their findings or else nobody will ever see their research. Journals that are considered respected are all Western, and it is no secret that they are biased against researchers and scientists in developing countries. Scientists have developed a way to rank journals depending on how often the articles published in them are cited by researchers.

   In the late 1990s, the US government came out with a landmark initiative in the name of PubMed. It is a huge database of all biomedical research in any part of the world and it allows scientists at least a quick look at the research without them having to spend hundreds of hours in libraries and manually trawling through it. The power of the Internet was used and the laborious task of bibliographical search reduced to the click of a button. Despite many advantages and ease of access, PubMed is an American database and does not include thousands of journals from around the world. Unsurprisingly, a large number of Indian journals are not in it. (A few are, though). This basically means that this research will never be visible to researchers in India and abroad. As a result, these articles will never be cited and this means Indian journals will continue to be ascribed lower ranks. This systematic rigging of research reputation probably goes on in other walks of life too but I can only talk about biomedical sciences with any degree of authority, as I did launch a web platform to try to address some of these weaknesses. (Again, please note my competing interests here.)

What I don't understand is why Indians always feel this need to look up to the West. Yes, the quality of our research is poor today, but it will remain so if we don't consciously address the systematic flaws therein. With the vast pool of software talent available in our country, I am confident we can create an IndMed (or give it any other name you like), which includes all peer-reviewed scientific literature, including that which has gone through post-publication peer review, a system that our organization (Webmed Limited, UK) was the first one globally to propose for biomedical sciences. The proposed database will include all the journals covered by PubMed and the many thousands of other journals it does not. In one stroke, this will correct all imbalances in visibility of scientific literature.

Secondly, the current system of ranking of academics, journals and even universities is somewhat flawed for it relies too much on the citation of research. This system of 'Impact Factor' was developed by an academic called Eugene Garfield in the 1970s and is still operated by a private company called

Thomson Reuters. Though a citation of research is important, it is not the only measure of its significance. It is a measure of the controversy or 'noise' a research piece generates rather than the contribution it makes. It is a flawed measure but it has stuck around for good as academics like to measure each other and this is the only measure they have traditionally had. However, newer measures for ranking are being developed (ResearchGate, a social media platform for researchers has developed one) and there is no reason why we can't develop an Indian measure that reflects Indian realities, goes beyond citation metrics, and probably includes 'Altmetrics' (a range of new metrics being developed to assess impact of research).

If we don't take these steps and also make our academic institutions autonomous and financially self-sufficient, where they can also take in students from around the globe and charge sustainable fees from students, we will continually lag in the academic race. And that sets the scene for the overall state of society.

10. **The Role of the Media:** In many respects, the media is already doing a good job of highlighting what is wrong with the medical profession and it must continue to do so. At the same time, certain sections of Indian media stand accused of catering to the masses. Yes, newspapers need to sell and channels need viewers but the media also has a responsibility towards shaping public opinion on important matters. For example, we need bigger focus in India on science and health charities as opposed to religious charities. Media could also bring to light instances of public sector incompetence (and not just corruption) more often. Currently, there is something of

an obsession in the media with trivia concerning politicians and celebrities. In a mature society, the kind that India aspires to be, this will need to change.

It is impossible to cover the entire edifice of Indian health care in one small book and to pretend that I have come even close to doing this would be a preposterous claim. Likewise, to claim that I have understood all the challenges our health service faces and know the solutions needed to fix it would probably indicate the same arrogance I detest in our bureaucrats and politicians. This books aims at opening up a discussion. It is an admission of a problem and an attempt at a collective discourse for a better tomorrow. Let us make a start.

Appendix 1

Hippocratic Oath

I swear by Apollo Physician, by Asclepius, by Health, by Heal-all, and by all the Gods and Goddesses, making them witnesses, that I will carry out, according to my ability and judgment, this oath and this indenture.

To regard my teacher in this art as equal to my parents; to make him partner in my livelihood, and when he is in need of money to share mine with him, to consider his offspring equal to my brothers; to teach them this art; if they require to learn it, without fee or indenture; and to impart precept, oral instruction, and all the other learning, to my sons, to the sons of my teacher, and to pupils who have signed the indenture and sworn obedience to the physicians' Law, but to none other. I will use treatment to help the sick according to my ability and judgment, but I will never use it to injure or wrong them. I will not give poison to anyone though asked to do so, nor will I suggest such a plan. Similarly, I will not give a pessary to a woman to cause abortion. But in purity and in holiness, I will guard my life and my art. I will not use the knife on sufferers from stone, but I will give place to such as are craftsmen therein.

Into whatsoever houses I enter, I will do so to help the sick, keeping myself free from all intentional wrongdoing and harm, especially from fornication with woman or man, bond or free.

Whatsoever in the course of practice I see or hear (or even outside my practice in social intercourse) that ought never to be published abroad, I will not divulge, but will consider such things to be holy secrets.

Now if I keep this oath and break it not, may I enjoy honour, in my life and art, among all men for all time; but if I transgress and forswear myself, may the opposite befall me.

Modern Oath

At the time of registration, each applicant shall be given a copy of the following declaration by the Registrar concerned and the applicant shall read and agree to abide by the same:

- I solemnly pledge myself to consecrate my life to the service of humanity.
- Even under threat, I will not use my medical knowledge contrary to the laws of humanity.
- I will maintain the utmost respect for human life from the time of conception.
- I will not permit considerations of religion, nationality, race, party politics or social standing to intervene between my duty and my patient.
- I will practise my profession with conscience and dignity.
- The health of my patient will be my first consideration.
- I will respect the secrets which are confined in me.
- I will give to my teachers the respect and gratitude which is their due.
- I will maintain by all means in my power, the honour and noble traditions of the medical profession.
- I will treat my colleagues with all respect and dignity.

- I shall abide by the code of medical ethics as enunciated in the Indian Medical Council (Professional Conduct, Etiquette and Ethics) Regulations 2002.
- I make these promises solemnly, freely and upon my honour.

Appendix 2

Adopted by the 2nd General Assembly of the World Medical Association, Geneva, Switzerland, September 1948

and amended by the 22nd World Medical Assembly, Sydney, Australia, August 1968

and the 35th World Medical Assembly, Venice, Italy, October 1983

and the 46th WMA General Assembly, Stockholm, Sweden, September 1994

and editorially revised by the 170th WMA Council Session, Divonne-les-Bains, France, May 2005

and the 173rd WMA Council Session, Divonne-les-Bains, France, May 2006

At the time of being admitted as a member of the medical profession:

I SOLEMNLY PLEDGE to consecrate my life to the service of humanity;

I WILL GIVE to my teachers the respect and gratitude that is their due;

I WILL PRACTISE my profession with conscience and dignity;

THE HEALTH OF MY PATIENT will be my first consideration;

I WILL RESPECT the secrets that are confided in me, even after the patient has died;

I WILL MAINTAIN by all the means in my power, the honour and the noble traditions of the medical profession;

MY COLLEAGUES will be my sisters and brothers;

I WILL NOT PERMIT considerations of age, disease or disability, creed, ethnic origin, gender, nationality, political affiliation, race, sexual orientation, social standing or any other factor to intervene between my duty and my patient;

I WILL MAINTAIN the utmost respect for human life;

I WILL NOT USE my medical knowledge to violate human rights and civil liberties, even under threat;

I MAKE THESE PROMISES solemnly, freely and upon my honour.

Acknowledgements

I would, first of all, like to thank my parents who despite very limited means at their disposal provided my sister and me with the best upbringing possible. From an early age, we were taught to step back and look at the broader picture when faced with difficult situations and be optimistic in the face of all adversity. It would seem clichéd to talk about your mother when thinking of the most profound influences in your life but I can't think of anyone else who has shaped my thoughts and personality more. I do not know of a wiser or more courageous woman. She instilled in me the importance of working hard with a resolute will from a very young age and, and the courage to fight for what you believe in. I would like to think those qualities endure and give me the strength to deal with every challenge that life periodically throws at me.

With his idealism and unwavering faith, my father was always going to find the world of business difficult but this did not deter him into instilling those values in us. He led by example where truth and honesty were more than mere words; they were the guiding principles of our lives. I will admit it hasn't exactly been easy safeguarding those values but it has nonetheless been very fulfilling.

Throughout my early years, I treated my little sister as my responsibility almost as if this was the payback for her almost devotional love and respect for me. It was difficult to get accustomed to the fact that she could grow into the independent and talented woman that she has. Our bond goes beyond what words are able to express.

During my school days, Dr Hridaya Narayana Upadhyay at Shree Jain Vidyalaya, Kolkata, was instrumental in teaching me not only the nuances of biology but also English language.

I am further indebted to all my teachers at Calcutta Medical College and Postgraduate Institute of Medical Education and Research, Chandigarh, for ensuring that my medical education went beyond textbooks. Professors S.K. Maitra, S.M. Bose, J.D. Wig, and many others ensured that care and compassion were as much a part of my basic medical education as the rigorous education and training. I don't know what they saw in me but they obviously spotted me for further personal mentoring and support for which I can only express utmost gratitude. If I have achieved anything at all the credit is theirs to take. All the shortcomings are no doubt mine and mine alone.

I have been very lucky at every stage of my life to have friends who not only have stood by me but also helped me learn and progress. Abhijit Bal and Navin Khattry will have to take most of the credit for getting rid of my thick accent and giving me the encouragement and confidence to read, write, and speak in English. Deepak Kejariwal and Siddhartha Gupta deserved to be thanked for enduring hundreds of hours of sometimes illogical discussions with me on various topics. I have always had a special relationship with Ajay Malviya which cannot be belittled by thanking him.

I have to also thank dozens of my other friends, previous and current colleagues, and many others who have provided me with a unique insights into the contemporary medical practice and the state of Indian health care. Vikash Agarwal, Rahul Saraf, Sanjay

Gupta, Chetan Parmar and so many others have selflessly shared anecdotes of experiences that form the backbone of this book. There are many others who cannot be mentioned here without compromising their positions as they still work in India.

I would also like to thank Rajesh Barnwal of India Medical Times, who not only encouraged me to write but went on to give me a regular column, The Antagonizer, on his rapidly growing web platform.

None of this, however, would have happened if Debasri Rakshit of HarperCollins had not asked me to write this book. She is sincere and dedicated to perfection. Her tact while dealing with difficult issues have not gone unnoticed, and her detached perspective is a huge asset for a first-time author. The editorial team, especially, Shreya Punj have done a remarkable job and improved the quality of writing.

Kush deserves to be thanked for letting me work on the book even during the holidays. For a ten-year-old boy, he has the most remarkable emotional quotient. I hope he can put his intelligence and ability to relate to others to good use.

Finally, and most importantly, Shalini, my wife is the reason this book could actually be written. Her faith in my ability is more than mine, and her talent for knowing the right from the wrong almost unique. She has sacrificed a lot to see me grow professionally. She works very hard on a daily basis to ensure that Kush and I can return to a loving home day after day. From managing finances, maintaining relationship with our huge circle of friends and family, and looking after Kush and me, in addition to a full-time job as an accomplished software engineer; she does it all with such grace. I could not find a better, more understanding, and more intelligent person to spend my life with.

Bibliography

1. http://www.wma.net/
2. Debbarma, J., Gupta, N., Aggarwal, N.K., 'Consumer Protection Act: Blessing or Curse to Medical Profession?', *Delhi Psychiatry Journal*, Volume XII (2), 2009, New Delhi
3. Nagral, S., 'General Practice: Some Thoughts', *Indian Journal of Medical Ethics*, Volume 10(2), 2002, New Delhi
4. Sachan, D., 'Tackling Corruption in Indian Medicine', *The Lancet*, Volume 382, 16 November 2013, London
5. Kale, P.A., 'An Objective Look at "Cut-practice" in the Medical Profession', *Indian Journal of Medical Ethics*, Volume IV, 1996, New Delhi
6. Balarajan, Y., Selvaraj, S., Subramanian, S.V., 'Healthcare and Equity in India', *The Lancet*, Volume 377, 2011, London
7. Pai, S.A., 'Unkind Cuts', *Indian Journal of Medical Ethics*, Volume 8(3): 90, 2000, New Delhi
8. Kaushik, S.P., 'Ethics in Surgical Practice: An Indian Viewpoint', *National Medical Journal of India*, Volume 15(1): 34-36, 2002, New Delhi
9. Berger, D., 'Corruption Ruins the Doctor-patient Relationship in India', The *BMJ*, Volume 348: g3169, 2014, London
10. http://www.bbc.co.uk
11. Gadre, A., 'India's Private Health Care Sector Treats Patients as Revenue Generators', The *BMJ*, Volume 350: h826, 2015, London
12. McCarthy, M., 'US Doctors Say Unnecessary Tests and Procedures are a Serious Concern', The BMJ, Volume 348: g3098, 2014, London
13. Roy, A., Madhiwalla, N., Pai, S.A., 'Drug Promotional Practices in Mumbai: A Qualitative Study', *Indian Journal of Medical Ethics*, Volume 4(2): 8-10, 2014, New Delhi

14. Waheed, K., Jaleel, M., Laeequddin M., 'Prescription loyalty behavior of physicians: an empirical study in India', *International Journal of Pharmaceutical and Healthcare Marketing*, Volume 5 (4): 279-98, 2011, United Kingdom
15. Kumar, S., 'Healthcare is among the Most Corrupt Services in India', The *BMJ*, Volume 326:10, 2003, London
16. Berger, D., 'Corruption Ruins the Doctor-Patient Relationship in India', The *BMJ*, Volume 348: g3169, 2014, London
17. Das, J., Holla, A., Das, V., Mohanan, M., Tabak, D., Chan, B., 'In Urban and Rural India, A Standardized Patient Study Showed Low Levels of Provider Training and Huge Quality Gaps', *Health Affiliated*, Volume 31(12): 2774-84, 2012, Millwood
18. Chaudhury, N., Hammer, J., Kremer, M., Muralidharan, K., Rogers, F.H., 'Missing in Action: Teacher and Health Worker Absence in Developing Countries', *Journal of Economic Perspectives*, Volume 20(1): 91-116, 2002, USA
19. Das, J., Hammer, J., Leonard, K., 'The Quality of Medical Advice in Low-income Countries', *Journal of Economic Perspectives*, Volume 22(2): 93-114, 2008, USA
20. Mudur, Ganapati, 'India Decides to Train Non-Medical Rural Health Care Providers', The *BMJ*, Volume 340: c817, 2010, London
21. Chatterjee, C., Srinivasan, V., 'Ethical Issues in Health Care Sector in India', *IIMB Management Review*, Volume 25(1): 49-62, 2013, Bengaluru
22. Garg, P., Nagpal, J., 'A Review of Literature to Understand the Complexity of Equity, Ethics and Management for Achieving Public Health Goals in India', *Journal of Clinical Diagnosis and Research*, Volume 8(2): 1-6, 2014, New Delhi
23. Anand, K., Kapoor, S.K., Pandav, C.S., 'Cost Analysis of a Primary Health Centre in Northern India', *National Medical Journal of India*, Volume 6(4): 160-3, 1993, New Delhi
24. Varatharajan, D., Thankappan, R., Jayapalan, S., 'Assessing the Performance of Primary Health Centres Under Decentralized Government in Kerala', *Health Policy Plan*, Volume 19(1): 41-51, January 2004, New Delhi